Deric Longden was born in Chesterfield in 1936 and married Diana Hill in 1957. They had two children, Sally and Nicholas. After various jobs he took over a small factory making lingerie, but he began writing and broadcasting in the 1970s and before long was writing regularly for programmes like *Does He Take Sugar?* and broadcasting on *Woman's Hour*, most of his work being closely based on his own experience. The demands made on him by Diana's illness, subsequently believed to be a form of ME, forced him to sell the factory, and since then he has devoted himself to writing, broadcasting, lecturing and after-dinner speaking. *Diana's Story*, published in 1989 some years after Diana's death, is a bestseller. His second and third books, *Lost For Words* and *The Cat Who Came In From the Cold*, are also available in Corgi paperback. Deric Longden married the writer Aileen Armitage in 1990 and now lives in Huddersfield.

Also by Deric Longden

LOST FOR WORDS
THE CAT WHO CAME IN FROM THE COLD

and published by Corgi Books

DIANA'S STORY

Deric Longden

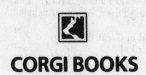

CORGI BOOKS

DIANA'S STORY
A CORGI BOOK 0 552 13944 0

Originally published in Great Britain by Bantam Press

PRINTING HISTORY
Bantam Press edition published 1989
Corgi edition published 1990
Corgi edition reprinted 1991
Corgi edition reprinted 1993
Corgi edition reissued 1993

This book is set in 11/13 pt. Bembo by Goodfellow & Egan
Cambridge Ltd.

Corgi Books are published by Transworld Publishers Ltd.,
61–63 Uxbridge Road, Ealing, London W5 5SA,
in Australia by Transworld Publishers (Australia) Pty. Ltd.,
15–25 Helles Avenue, Moorebank, NSW 2170, and in New
Zealand by Transworld Publishers (N.Z.) Ltd.,
3 William Pickering Drive, Albany, Auckland.

Printed and bound in Great Britain by
BPCC Paperbacks Ltd
Member of BPCC Ltd

1

'What have you done with Fred's hands?'

I pushed her gently away from me, to lift her left buttock about an inch or so, and polished it with the loofah.

'They're on the radiator in the kitchen.'

'They'll melt.'

'No, they won't – it's only just on.'

I eased her towards me and polished the right buttock. My rolled up sleeve gradually unfurled and sank beneath the water.

'Sod it.'

'You always do that.'

'I know.'

'You ought to roll them up properly – not just a couple of turns.'

'Robert Redford only turns them up twice.'

'He doesn't have to wash his wife's bum.'

I dried everything that was sticking out of the water – lifting Diana out of the bath was hard enough without her being wet and soapy – and then I slipped the towel under her right arm for extra purchase. She breathed in to make herself lighter, and I set my knees and waited for the pain in my groin.

*

I sat her in the chair and dried her feet.

'I should have painted my toenails. He'll want to look at my legs.'

'We haven't time – he'll be here in half an hour.' I rolled up my soggy sleeve. Just a couple of turns, like Robert Redford.

'I wish he wasn't coming. What if he thinks I'm putting it on? I wish I felt poorly.'

I dried her legs and her tummy. Her breasts and back were heavy with perspiration. Pain always made her sweat. I bathed her with a warm flannel and dried her once more.

'How can he think you're putting it on? Just don't try to be so bloody brave when he comes.'

'I can't help it, I am bloody brave.'

'You're bloody awkward as well.'

We prepared for our twelve-yard marathon back to the bedroom. My left hand under her left elbow, my right arm around her waist. Her left leg was the one that refused to work – the right leg was coming out in sympathy. My right leg, hard up against her left, served as a crutch and we slowly Jake-the-Pegg'ed along the landing and into the room. We both swung around on our heels, a well-practised movement that would surely have brought a five-point-eight from the judges, and then crashed backwards on to the bed.

'Which nightie do you want?'

'Which do you think?'

'I don't know – they're all disgusting.'

I produced a little black number from the drawer. Split up the sides to the hip and from the neck down to the waist, it was difficult to work out which way up it was supposed to be.

'You've got it the wrong way up.'

I turned it over.

'Oh no, you hadn't – what about that one?'

That one was a bright scarlet with a sheer lace bodice. Four wisps of satin formed the skirt and it had cost my mother a fortnight's pension. For a seventy-two-year-old woman my mother has a rare taste in nighties. 'It's upper-class tart this one,' she had said as she had given the box to Diana.

We decided on the scarlet on the basis that the others were indecent and not at all suitable for a doctor who was coming to assess whether or not the cripple was indeed crippled.

Diana pointed her arms at the ceiling and I lowered the nightie over her head. I managed to screw it down only as far as her breasts – again she was lathered with the sweat of pain.

After another warm flannel and an all-over dab with the bath towel we eased the nightie into place and then, after a pillow-pluffing session, she was sitting up in bed, a gentle smile on her lovely face.

'I do look decent, don't I?'

Not for Diana the sensible brushed nylon from Marks & Spencers or a voluminous cotton nightshirt with Garfield grinning out at the world. Nature was attacking her on all fronts and, in hospital and out, her femininity needed boosting with nylon, lace and narrow straps. Young doctors, housemen, who would peel flannelette from the pink flesh that lay on a hospital bed whilst still dreaming of the bacon sandwich they had left in the rest room, would find their mouths becoming dry as they removed a black strap from a tanned shoulder. It was a good thing – it evened things up. It transformed 'bed fourteen' into a woman, which is all you can ask for in hospital.

She looked down at the lace bodice. 'Can you see my nipples?'

'No,' I lied, and then the front door bell sounded.

'It's him – I'm not ready – what's his name?'

I grabbed the letter from the bedside table.

'Dr Harvey – don't panic – he's probably very nice.'

I'd reached the bedroom door when she shouted.

'Fred's hands – I need Fred's hands.'

'I'll bring them up – I must let him in.'

As I tumbled down the stairs the bell was accompanied by the steady thump of fist upon door. He might be 'nice', but patience wasn't his long suit and he sounded as though he'd brought an axe with him. I tugged the door open and the postman fell in.

'You took your time,' he grumbled.

'I thought you were the doctor.'

'Leave him waiting that long and he'll bugger off – now then.'

He fanned six letters out in his hand. This was our daily ritual. The postman was a would-be writer – he loved to see envelopes emblazoned with 'BBC' or '*Woman's World*'. He couldn't bear just to shove them through the letterbox – he had to see what was in them.

He handed me number one.

'Rates, final demand. Don't worry, they've all got 'em in this street, they never pay on time round here.'

He sorted out number two.

'Bank statement . . . and here's a postcard from your lad. From Yarmouth – "Love, Nick and Jo." Has he gone with the Henshaws' lass, then?'

'Yes.'

'I suppose her mother knows about it?'

'Yes, of course she does – can I have the others?'

He waved a large brown envelope at me.

'*She* magazine. That's a rejection, that is, and there's two from the BBC, one local and one from London. Probably cheques.'

I took them from him.

'Aren't you going to open them?'

'Later,' I said. 'The doctor will be here any minute.'

'Right.' He looked disappointed. 'I'll be off, then. Wife said she heard you on "Woman's Hour" yesterday – said you weren't as funny as usual.'

I squeezed the door shut behind him and slipped into the kitchen where Fred's hands were drying.

Diana's hands were clawed. Something – God knows what – made her fingers twist until the nails bit into her palms and then she would have them forcibly straightened, often until they broke and had to be reset. Fred's hands were designed to slow the process down.

Fred was in charge of the Plaster Theatre at the Hallamshire Hospital in Sheffield, and his creations were works of wonder. Diana had two sets for each hand. One had a plaster cast that covered the outer arm from just below the elbow to the knuckles. Then four great metal arches leapt out of the back of the hands and hovered above the fingers like the bridge over the River Kwai. From each arch there was suspended an elastic band with a little upside-down saddle to take a finger. This stretched her fingers as straight as they would go – the thumb had its own little plaster cast. Set two were perfect casts of her inner arm, wrist and palms, and carried on to take the weight of her fingers, which were lashed in place with Velcro.

Thanks to Fred and his loving expertise, they gave Diana comfort and cut down the visits to the breaker's yard, although eventually the force that twisted her fingers would triumph over Fred's wire and plaster and his creation would crack and crumble.

'Never mind – we can rebuild her,' Fred would tell me as he bent Diana's fingers into a new contraption. 'Always remember, love – this is going to hurt you a lot more than it hurts me.'

Fred's hands were dry. It was my job to remove the biro marks, gravy and nail varnish with Dabitoff, and then the general grime with Ajax liquid. Some people clean the front doorstep when important people are about to call, others have their hair done. Diana had her 'hands' shampooed.

We fitted them in place and their whiteness was a credit to me. Another dab with the flannel and then we sat – waiting.

'Did I tell you I interviewed a woman who slept with her goat at Chatsworth Show?'

'Yes.'

'She was cleaning it all the time we talked.'

'So you said.'

'She even pushed a Johnson's cotton wool bud up its bottom.'

'Can you see his car yet?'

The next ten minutes flew past like a fortnight. Dr Patrick Harvey's visit was important, to say the least. It would determine, among other things, whether or not we would eat in the future. We had applied for Day and Night Attendance Allowance and the Married Woman's Invalidity Pension. The two together added up to over fifty pounds a week, and God knows we needed it. Over the past five years my business had almost bled to death – now it had a gaping wound. My radio and newspaper work had also suffered. I could never guarantee to be anywhere at a certain time, because Diana might need me. Producers and editors had been very good – for a time. They had their own problems.

Dr Harvey was to determine whether or not Diana qualified – whether she was sufficiently disabled to require day and night attendance.

I had, fleetingly, considered amputation just to be on the safe side.

Diana snapped on the television. Mavis Nicholson was halfway through one of her long, convoluted questions.

'Get on with it,' ordered Diana, but Mavis ignored her and continued to unwrap her words like so many sticky sweets.

'Right,' said Diana, and Mavis's image withered and disappeared down the tube.

The doorbell rang again.

I had plans for Dr Harvey – I wanted a couple of minutes alone with him before he marched upstairs to Diana. He had to know that she could absorb pain like a middleweight champion – that she would never say that she felt ill to anyone but me. Her smile never fooled me – I could tell from her eyes – but she could run rings around a newcomer who didn't know her. She wouldn't whinge for fifty pounds a week.

Just a couple of minutes alone, that's all I needed – I was well rehearsed.

I opened the door.

'Sign here, please – they're out next door.'

This was another part of my new life – taking in mail order ironing boards for people who worked normal hours, and then delivering them after five o'clock. I stacked it in the kitchen with the Gascoignes' toaster and the Spencers' wok, and made a mental note to nip round and give David Croft his free soil-testing kit from the *Reader's Digest* – he'd be thrilled to bits with that.

'I presume Mrs Longden is upstairs?'

It had to be Dr Harvey. Tall, grey, handsome and distinguished, he would have made an ideal partner for Dr Kildare.

'Yes – could I have a . . . ?'

He was halfway upstairs already and I trailed behind him.

'In here?'

'Yes – if I could just . . .'

He was in, and I couldn't. I followed him in through the door and he turned.

'Thank you.'

I was dismissed. Diana sat up in bed and beamed at him, looking perky and bright, her nipples standing to attention through the scarlet lace.

Dr Harvey produced a form from his briefcase.

'And how are you?'

'Fine, thank you.'

I groaned, and went to plug in the percolator.

*

13

I gave them fifteen minutes and then appeared with three cups of coffee – the best cups.

Dr Harvey sat on the edge of the bed, his briefcase acting as a desk upon his knee. His manner had changed to one of concern, and Diana had that brightness about her that told me that her reserves of energy were about to burn out.

He paused, with his pen above the paper.

'Your left leg is paralysed, isn't it?'

'No.'

'No?'

'Not really – I can get about the bedroom if I lean on the dressing table and then sit on the end of the bed and then swing my leg and reach out for the . . .'

'Your leg is paralysed, isn't it?'

'Well, it's numb at the moment but . . .'

'For God's sake, woman – your leg is paralysed, isn't it?'

Diana looked at me. She looked wounded. She was always going to get better – they would find what was causing it all and cut it out. Or they would discover that she was allergic to something or other and it would all go away. If she stopped eating butter her fingers would straighten. If she stopped eating white bread her legs would work again. They'd find out before long – if she stopped eating meat the pain would disappear. She couldn't be paralysed – that was too permanent. She needed hope.

'Yes.'

'Thank God for that.' Dr Harvey began to write, and Diana and I looked at one another in silence. He stopped writing.

'You need help, my girl – not just medical help. Your head is too full of questions – you need answers.'

She began, slowly at first, and then it all came in a rush. Her frustration with the medical profession who would tell her nothing and who, worse still, wouldn't listen. The consultants who promised results and who, when they failed to come up with any, were never there to explain their failure as she was sent home. She could handle the pain – she just wanted to know what was wrong with her body.

He listened, talking gently every now and then and, as her fire burned out, he took her hand.

'I'll leave my card. If you need to talk, just ring me any time, day or night, it doesn't matter.'

She was to spend many hours with Pat Harvey, and not one second of them would be wasted.

I saw him to the door.

'Take care of her, and see she rings me if she needs me.'

Diana lay back in the bed, her energy spent and the pain crowding in on her.

'He was nice.'

'He was very nice.' I gave her a sip of cold coffee.

'I'm paralysed.'

'Only bits of you, love – some bits are perfect.'

'Do you think I'm going to die?'

'No.'

'I wouldn't mind.'

'I would.'

She flicked on the television – Mavis Nicholson had gone home.

'I know, let's do something together.'

'All right, what?'

'Let's clean out the garage. You put your old jeans on and I'll lie here and think you through it.'

'OK, but you mustn't overdo it.'

'I won't – I promise.'

2

The phone rang at seven-thirty a.m. I think I answered it around twenty-five to eight.

Diana had had a bad night – a three-bath night to ease the pain – and the phone took some finding. My mother, however, is persistent. She will often dial a number and then go and feed the cat, but she was ready and waiting when I eventually made contact.

'Deric? I've lost my voice,' she told me in ringing tones.

'Can you remember where you had it last?'

'I think I got a chill when we went round Longleat.'

I had forgotten about Longleat – she had gone with the Autumn Club.

'Did you see any lions?'

'One was playing with a squirrel, and the other one had a limp.'

I could have sworn they had more than two lions at Longleat, but maybe I was mistaken.

'I told a big monkey off for hitting a little monkey, and we saw a deaf giraffe.'

There was no way I was going to ask my mother how she could tell that the giraffe was deaf – not at that time in the morning.

17

'We saw a pair of rhinos called René and Renata – they weren't as tall as I thought they would be, but Mr Eckersley said they were standing in a ditch.'

I couldn't think of a thing to say, and my mother hates silences.

'Anyway,' she said briskly, 'I'm ever so busy – what was it you wanted?'

'You rang me.'

'Did I?'

'You do every morning.'

She thought for a moment, trying to remember what it was she wanted to tell me.

So I asked, 'How is the cat?'

'I'm worried about him – I think he's going deaf. Whenever I talk to him he just ignores me.'

'Perhaps it's only a temporary condition – whilst you've lost your voice.'

'I never thought of that,' she said. 'You're probably right – and that would account for the giraffe.'

'Of course,' I agreed, and she rang off happily.

Breakfast was the easy meal of the day – I could handle breakfast. A slice of toast and a cup of coffee for me, and the same for Diana later on. Nick always prepared his own particular feast – a couple of Weetabix doing the breaststroke in a pint and a half of milk. He'd chase them around the pyrex bowl, harrying them, until they finally gave up and disintegrated. At weekends, when he had more time, he would pursue Farley's rusks for a change. They were made of sterner stuff and often put up quite a fight.

When Sally was at home she would appear in the doorway, a slim, elegant figure in her Laura Ashley nightdress and rugby socks, bearing on a tray her breakfast of cold boiled potatoes, jelly, condensed milk and a stick of celery. She would munch away in silence – until she came to the celery.

The kids had been wonderful; like the Farley's rusks, they were made of sterner stuff. Sally had been fifteen and Nick just two years younger when Diana first became ill five years earlier, and they had pitched in like troupers.

Sally took over the running of the shops for long periods, studying between customers. Nick would call in on his way home from school: 'You go and have a coffee, Sal – I'll take over.'

Then, at closing time as I called to pick them up, I would wait at the door, out of sight, and eavesdrop as he handled a customer.

'The tie-side briefs are very popular – if you're worried about the tie showing through your skirt, my sister wears them all the time and she doesn't have any trouble.'

'What colours have you got?'

'All the pastel shades plus black, white and red.'

'I've never had red.'

'Now they do show through your skirt, especially

19

in the summer – doesn't look very attractive. What about skintone?'

'Yes, all right – and I'll have a pair of white as well.'

'Thank you.' The till chinked. 'You want to get your husband to buy you the red ones for Christmas. Husbands always buy either black or red, and we've got suspender belts and garters to match.'

Not bad for a thirteen-year-old rugby player. Now he was eighteen, and if the postman was surprised that Mrs Henshaw would let him take her sixteen-year-old daughter off to Yarmouth for a week – then I was astonished. I wouldn't have trusted him as far as I could throw him.

After a second cup of coffee, a cup of tea and another coffee I was ready for whatever the day had to throw at me.

No need to go into the factory today. I had three jobs. A lingerie factory to run, the writing – which now earned me more than the factory – and Diana, who was more important than the other two put together and who took up most of my time.

Diana's shops had been a natural extension of the factory. She had started with lingerie parties and quickly outgrown them. Then came the first shop in Chesterfield and a second in Matlock, and a sideways move into high fashion. Now the shops had been sold. At first Diana had tried to run them from the bed in which she was spending more and more time. I spent much of my time interpreting her ideas and seeing that they were carried out. Sally's efforts were heroic – but it was Diana the customers wanted to see, and it was her flair and enthusiasm that made the shops buzz with life. Without her – and her knack of filling the racks with taste and colour and the shelves with fun and fashion – the customers began to go elsewhere. We employed a professional buyer who, unfortunately, was stuck in a crimplene time-lock, and thousands of pounds later the shops were quietly put to sleep.

My factory was also nodding off. I needed to spend all my time there, but more often than not I would drive in, make my excuses and leave.

'I'll try and be back by two o'clock – it depends how Diana is. Try and find something to do if I'm not. The windows could do with cleaning.'

'We'll see you tomorrow, then.' The girls knew me well.

It was losing hundreds of pounds a week, but Diana needed me more.

'Why don't you employ a nurse?' asked my accountant.

It was a fair question, and I'm not sure that my answer was good enough, but I just couldn't bring myself to care by proxy.

Diana needed *me* – not an efficient substitute in a starched apron. All right, a nurse could bath her, deal with her blackouts and half carry her to the toilet – but I could do it with love, and Diana needed love much more than she needed efficiency, pain killers and Valium.

'Why don't you sell the factory?'

'I can't, it's my living.'

Besides, who would want to buy a business that was not so much running downhill as tumbling head over heels?

'Close it down, then.'

'I'd love to – but I should have to sell my house to cover the redundancy payments.'

If Joseph Heller had invented 'Catch 22', then I had invented 'Catch 22½' and it was most unpleasant. I had an ulcer, and so had my ulcer. But I also had Diana, and who could tell when I might lose her – certainly not the doctors, who didn't even know what was wrong with her. In the meantime I was going to spend as much time as I could with her.

When she awoke, Diana couldn't move. I sat on the edge of the bed and massaged her fingers gently – very gently. It was a necessary agony, but they had to be made to move. After a night stuck in Fred's contraptions they had locked, but at least they hadn't clawed. Once they had clawed we couldn't do anything with them. After a quarter of an hour I began to work on her legs and then, forming her into the shape of a question mark, went to run a bath. A hot bath was her only refuge from pain – this was to be her fourth since midnight. It was half past eight in the morning.

22

I squatted on the bathroom floor reading *Woman's World* whilst Diana hunted for the soap.

'There isn't any soap.'

I decided to have a little search round, deep down in the bubbly depths of the bath – you have to take your pleasures where you find them, don't you? I only wish I had rolled up my dressing gown sleeve first.

'Ouch!' yelped Diana.

'Sorry.'

'Have a look in the airing cupboard, there might be some in there – and cut your fingernails tonight.'

There wasn't any soap where you would normally expect to find soap in the airing cupboard, and so I wiggled my hand through the wooden slats to see if the odd bar had slipped down behind the tank and found my thumb stuck in the top of a hot water bottle.

I drifted back into the bathroom. 'There's only a soap on a rope,' I said. It was a football that I had been given for Christmas the year England won the World Cup, and all the pattern had worn off.

'Isn't there any in the kitchen?' asked Diana.

'There's a tin of Swarfega.'

'I'll have the soap on a rope,' she decided, and I hung it around her wrist so that it couldn't escape.

Her fingers were too weak to hold a piece of soap for long, and she would drop it roughly fifteen times a bath.

'That's clever.' She was delighted. 'I shan't keep losing it now.'

I wasn't so enthusiastic – I enjoyed looking for it, it would hide in the most amazing places.

The hot water was working its short-lived miracle and drowning the pain. It would be back again in twenty minutes.

I tried to wring out my dressing gown sleeve in the sink but gave up and settled down again, stark naked, on the bathroom floor.

'What first attracted you to me?' I asked her.

'What makes you think I *am* attracted to you?'

'Well,' I said, 'you married me and you've stuck with me and you still accept expensive gifts from me.'

'What expensive gifts?' she wanted to know.

'That soap on a rope was mine originally,' I pointed out. 'Come on – don't be shy, just tell me what bit of my anatomy did you find so erotic that you felt you just had to have me?'

'Well,' she said thoughtfully, twirling the rope and cracking herself on the knee with the soap, 'I think that if I had ever thought that one day I would see you sitting on the bathroom floor reading a women's magazine with a hot water bottle stuck on your thumb – then perhaps I might have said no.'

'I can't seem to get it off,' I said, waving the hot water bottle up and down.

'Screw it,' said Diana.

'Pardon?'

'Screw it off,' she repeated. 'That's how the stopper comes out.'

She's very clever – she has an 'O' level in embroidery. I screwed it to the left and it slowly crept halfway up my arm.

'The other way,' she said impatiently, so I twisted it to the right and the hot water bottle fell lifeless to the floor.

'What were you saying about erotic bits and pieces?'

'It says here,' I said, pointing out the page, 'that women think that a man's best asset is a beautiful bum.'

'Does it?' she said.

'Yes – it says that bottoms are tops.'

'Oh,' she said.

I hate it when people refuse to carry on a conversation. I can't stand the silence and I talk even more rubbish than usual.

'They have a list of Britain's top ten bums here,' I went on. 'Sting the singer won it and Cliff Richard came sixth, and I'm only a bit older than Cliff Richard.'

'Are you asking me in your awkward, bumbling, roundabout way whether I think you have a good bottom or not?' She can read me like a book – one with large print and words of one syllable.

'No,' I protested. ' . . . Yes.'

'You have a very nice bottom,' she said, thoughtfully. 'Despite the ravages of the years it remains taut and cheeky and it's well rounded in a most understated manner.'

At that moment I knew exactly what a mini-skirted girl must feel like as she walks past a building site.

'Unfortunately,' said Diana – there's usually an 'unfortunately' with Diana – 'Unfortunately, even though you have a bottom that could be described as verging on the pert, it's not possible for you to spend your whole life with your back to me.'

'Ah,' I said, 'but there's more to this survey than that. Although thirty-nine per cent of the women said that they admired a beautiful bottom, another fifteen per cent said that slimness attracted them.'

'Well,' she said. 'You're certainly . . .'

'Slender,' I suggested.

'Scrawny,' she thought.

'Lean,' I offered.

'Spindly,' she countered.

'Spare?'

'More sort of scraggy.'

'Would you settle for wiry?' I asked, and so we settled for wiry. I think I would rather have been lean, but you have to be tall like Gary Cooper to qualify as lean, don't you?

'Now then,' I said. 'Thirteen per cent of the women in this survey admired a flat tummy – they said they found a flat tummy very sexy.'

I relaxed – my stomach has always born a strong

resemblance to Lincolnshire, that's one advantage we wiry types have.

'I've noticed,' said Diana, 'that recently you have had a little roll of fat creeping up round your tummy.'

I breathed in instinctively. 'There is not.'

'Put that magazine down and let's have a look.' I dropped the magazine to the floor.

'You're holding it in.'

'I'm not,' I protested through gritted teeth.

'You are – you're holding your breath.'

'Rubbish!' I told her, my lungs almost bursting.

'You're cheating,' she said, and lobbed the soap on a rope at me from the bath. I side-stepped and trod on the hot water bottle.

'Look,' Diana pointed out gleefully. 'Talk about pinch an inch – you could fondle a foot.'

My ego deflated in direct contrast to my waistline and lay quivering on the floor alongside the soap on a rope.

'If you really want to know what first attracted me to you,' said Diana, 'it was your smile.'

'Really?' My face split from side to side with delight and surprise.

'You have a lovely smile and your eyes are all crinkly around the edge.'

I smiled her a lovely smile. 'That's the nicest thing you've ever said,' I told her.

'It's true,' she told me. 'Do me a favour and make a pot of coffee.'

'Anything, my love,' I beamed at her.

'And Deric,' she added as I reached the bathroom door.

'Yes?'

'Take that silly grin off your face.'

3

The Citroën floated through Baslow and on towards Sheffield and the Royal Hallamshire Hospital. Diana floated in the passenger seat. The Citroën had been one of my better buys and it had replaced the Audi coupé which had, in its youth, belonged to Geoff Duke, the Isle of Man TT champion.

I had loved that car. It would throw itself around corners as though saying 'This is how Geoff used to do it', and it was noisy and raucous. The fact that it was, on occasions, overtaken by Minis and the odd Reliant Robin never diminished that love, because I knew that, if only I could harness the raw power of the machine and find a mechanic who could tune it properly, then I would leave them all wallowing in my wake.

I never did, but it *looked* fast, especially when parked, and it had a sun roof and I had never had one of those before. What it didn't have was a recognizable suspension system, and after any journey of over ten miles I would have to take a rest to allow my eyeballs to settle. Diana had to be nestled amidst a mountain of pillows, and still I would see her face tighten with pain at the slightest bump, pebble or hedgehog. It had to go, and John Lamb, the local

29

Porsche agent, found me the Citroën. It was an Athena with that wonderfully eccentric hydraulic suspension peculiar to Citroëns, and the colour was Mampoo. People would admire the car.

'That's nice. What colour is it – gold?'

'No, it's Mampoo.'

'Mampoo? It looks gold to me.'

'Yes, well – you know what daft names they think up nowadays.'

It was just a year later, as I retaxed the car, that I discovered that Mampoo was the prefix to the engine number. The colour was listed as gold.

Just a single cushion at the neck was all Diana needed in the Citroën, and twenty minutes later we pulled into the hospital car park.

Diana's medical history was bizarre, to say the least – everything was going wrong and nobody knew why. That was the most frustrating aspect of the whole business. It all seemed to spring from a fever – a sort of flu. The fever went but the exhaustion remained, and her arms and legs became weak and the fatigue took over her body. Then one day she had tried to get out of the car and her legs wouldn't work.

The use came back after a panicky half hour, but the pain had remained and grown steadily worse over the years until it was unmanageable. Then the hands had clawed, at times so badly that her arms followed suit, so that her elbows bent backwards over her shoulders and her hands pointed down her back. At such times a fever swept over her, then, as it left her, the hands and arms would return to normal – the hands just slightly more skeletal each time and the arms left just a little weaker.

It was at the Hallamshire Hospital that Diana had a biopsy performed on her left leg – just another test, a small piece of muscle to be removed from her thigh. Nothing much – they did dozens a week. She walked in by herself, albeit a little unsteadily, but afterwards she was never able to use that leg again.

Convalescing at home, the leg ballooned from ankle to thigh until the skin was translucent and a delicate shade of blue. Dr MacFarlane, our GP, was worried and he sent her back to the hospital. They had no idea why it was happening, but said it couldn't have anything to do with the biopsy.

'How do you know it has nothing to do with the biopsy if you have no idea why it is happening?'

'Well, it can't have.'

'Why can't it?'

'It just can't have.'

Several weeks and a hundred questions later the answers became more involved as more brilliant minds concerned themselves with the matter. But the answer always boiled down to: 'Well, it can't have.'

Eventually at such times the fury burns itself out, resignation sets in and energy is diverted to coping. For a layman, cross-examining a doctor who is on the defensive and retreating more and more into the sophistry of medical jargon is like discussing your Audi's big-end in Serbo-Croat with a Yugoslavian motor mechanic. In the end you say: 'Well, do what you can, then – will you?' and you thank him for his trouble. Doctors have a knack of proving everything to you – to their own satisfaction.

We always made a day of it at the Hallamshire. Diana would have four appointments. The first one of the day would be with the neurologist, the second with the Renal Unit (her kidneys, having had little attention thus far, were beginning to feel neglected and were demanding equal time). The third visit would be to the Hand Clinic and then, finally, on to the Plaster Theatre for Fred to check up on his handiwork.

'Where first?'

'Neurology – I want to get it over with.'

The difference in the atmosphere between the waiting area at the Hand Clinic and that at Neurology was remarkable. At the Hand Clinic customers were sprayed all over the corridor and in and out of little rooms off it. In addition to 'hands' there would be legs and backs and arms and heads, all fractured and waiting to be wheeled through other doors. Some would have fallen off roofs – others would have had roofs fall upon them. There would be football injuries, those struck a glancing blow by a passing truck and one woman, of blessed memory, who had broken her foot when a three-and-a-half-pound frozen chicken leapt out of the fridge and landed on it. But, apart from certain exceptions whose injuries were dreadful, there was an air of optimism about the place. Within weeks or months all would be well, and in the meantime the sympathy and admiration of friends was to be relished.

'What's happened to you?'

'This car ploughed into my motorbike.'

'Christ!'

'There's a steel pin right through the bone.'

'Bloody hell!'

'Doctor says it was one of the worst he's ever seen.'

'Good God! Can I have a go with your crutch?'

The novelty would wear off as the plaster cast grew grubby – but there was always that day ahead when all would be well again.

Not so in the Neurology Department. Many of those waiting were regulars. Husbands grown old to the point where lifting the wheelchair out of the boot was a daunting task. Wives who had hauled fifteen-stone husbands out of bed that morning, dressed and toileted them before wheeling them down the tiled corridors – they looked knackered and it was only eleven-thirty in the morning.

There would be children with wise faces who had experienced more pain and humiliation in their short lives than most adults ever did in theirs. No sharp anticipation of what the doctor might say this time

– it would be what he had said last time and the time before that.

'Yes. Well, I think we might try . . . er . . . er . . . might as well give it a shot.'

Spectacular cures for the masses are few and far between in neurology – they would be back in three months' time for a shot at something else. 'It's wonderful what they can do nowadays' would rarely be heard in here.

The air of resignation would be punctuated by a few bright faces – the newcomers.

'Excuse me – it's almost twenty to twelve, and my appointment was for ten-thirty.'

'We all are, love – we're all ten-thirties.'

Forty or so heads would nod in agreement, and the newcomer would settle down with an ancient *Country Life* advertising houses in Darlington at £7,500 and chrome bath taps at three shillings and sixpence a pair.

'Mrs Longden?'

The nurse at the open door ushered us into a bare room. A filing cabinet, an empty chair and a desk complete with young doctor flicking through a file roughly the size of a small fridge.

'I'll be with you in a moment – I'll just have a look through this.'

No consultant again. I suppose they can't be everywhere at once, but three months is a long time to wait to see yet another stand-in. It was a young woman with acne last time.

I plonked the wheelchair up against the desk and retired stage left to watch the proceedings.

The doctor 'Mmmm-mmmmmed' his way through Diana's case notes and then, turning his head through ninety degrees, he looked me straight in the eye and asked, 'How are her periods?'

'She's sitting right opposite you – why don't you ask her?'

There was nowhere the interview could go from there. Perhaps, had he been Jesus and had he cured her by a laying on of hands right there and then, he might just have scraped through. As it was, the white coat and stethoscope only thinly disguised a young man who was way out of his depth.

The case notes contained the results of tests from three London hospitals – the Royal Free, the Maudsley and the National in Queen Square, as well as the Hallamshire's own findings. To them all, Diana was still a mystery. He hadn't had a chance even to glance through the notes before Diana's wheelchair nosed its way into the office. In short – he hadn't a chance.

As the wheelchair bounced down the corridor I could see in Diana's rigid back all the rage and frustration – all the hurt and confusion that was welling up inside her. She was bright – she was intelligent. She didn't expect some miracle cure to emanate from these brief consultations, but these precious moments face to face with a neurologist were the only moments when she could discuss intelligently the questions that knotted up her mind as she lay,

35

week after week, in her bed. For days before the visit she would go through the questions in her mind – questions about *her* body, and if the answers were negative then so be it. It would make space for more questions until one day . . .

'The idiot – the bloody idiot.' Tears were running down her cheeks.

'Don't worry, love.'

'Does he think I need an interpreter to tell him about my periods?'

'We'll make an appointment to see the consultant privately.'

'The bloody idiot.'

'It'll only take a week.'

'We can't afford it.'

'Course we can.'

We would have to. The questions would go round and round in her mind until it jammed – it had happened before, and the consultant would see her at his home, privately. Anyway, he was a different man away from the hospital – more at ease, more time. He sat on the couch and talked and held her hand privately. It was only a matter of money.

I stopped the wheelchair at the reception desk. 'We have to make another appointment.'

'No – I'm not coming again. It's useless.'

The nurse raised her eyebrows, awaiting a decision.

'He's a big prick.'

36

The eyebrows raced up the nurse's forehead and froze.

'Can I make an appointment for . . . ?'

'He's the biggest – the most stupid – the biggest pr . . .'

'I'll ring you,' I told the nurse, and quickly shuffled Diana off down the corridor and around the corner.

' . . . ick in the world.'

'Feel better?'

'A bit.'

We passed through the main reception, down another corridor and into the Renal Unit. The waiting room was crowded.

'He wants castrating,' Diana announced to the assembled throng and the ladies parted, giving me plenty of elbow room and three chairs all to myself.

The nurses in the Renal Unit were bright and lively and shepherded by a sister who never seemed to forget a face or a name.

'Hullo, Diana – how are you, love?'

'Fine, thank you.'

They discussed kidneys at length and then moved on to holidays and feet. Nurses are preoccupied with feet. The younger ones with feet and fellas – the older ones simply with feet.

An old lady sank down in the chair next to me clutching a wad of purple lavatory paper.

'Do you mind if I sit next to you?'

'Not at all.'

'Only I sweat a lot, you see.'

'That must be uncomfortable.'

'After I've been up an hour, you could wring me vest out.'

We talked perspiration for some time, exploring several theories. One was that although she had gone through 'the change' twenty-five years ago, she wondered if it could be that again – only this time she was approaching it from a different direction.

I said I thought it was unlikely.

'My husband says I do it on purpose – you can't sweat on purpose, can you?'

We discussed vests. Did a thick vest, although it soaked up the perspiration admirably, tend to make you sweat more than a thin one?

'Just to be on the safe side I wear two – a thick one and a thin one.'

I had an idea. 'Have you thought of not wearing a vest at all?'

She snorted and fluttered her eyes, then, leaning across the front of me, said, 'He's cheeky, your husband, isn't he?'

'He's a little rascal,' agreed Diana, and took over the conversation.

Slowly we moved, chair by chair, towards the room where Mr Williams held court. He had a brisk but kindly manner. He was efficient and prepared to listen and explain. He had helped Diana a lot. She had a kidney infection that wouldn't go away. Antibiotics kept it at bay but wouldn't cure it – at its height it caused blackouts and delirium. In check, it was a bloody nuisance.

One by one the patients trooped into the office secretively palming little sample bottles of urine. My dual-vested neighbour had no such qualms. She held her sample up to the light.

'Just look at the colour of that.'

Diana and I admired it at a distance and then, for the second time that day –

'Mrs Longden.'

The sister wheeled Diana in to see Mr Williams and I pulled out a notebook. I had a radio piece to write for the morning and I jotted down one or two phrases. 'Do you mind if I sit next to you? Only I sweat a lot, you see.' 'Just look at the colour of that.'

My neighbour jogged my elbow. She held her urine sample aloft.

'Look – it's all clear.'

She shook the bottle vigorously.

'Look – now it's all cloudy.'

I wrote it down in my notebook.

The sister appeared in the doorway and came across to me.

'Can you come with me – Diana has blacked out again.'

I followed her into the room and I could see Diana in her wheelchair, her back to me and her head lolling on one shoulder. A nurse was talking to her through the mists and patting her face lightly.

It's always difficult to take over when you are in professional company, but I had done this so many times before and, sensibly, the nurses didn't object. I lifted her head gently until it was upright and waited. She could be brought round by shaking or shouting, but unless her head was held in a perfect line with her body then she would pass out again. I have no idea why.

We waited another minute or so and, as her breathing became heavier, she opened her eyes, gazed up at the anxious faces and smiled.

'What?'

'You passed out for a moment or so,' Mr Williams told her.

'Oh, I do that a lot,' said Diana as she tried to focus her eyes on the room. 'Deric knows what to do – I should get Deric if I were you.'

I was standing in front of her, holding her head in my hands.

'I'm here – don't worry.'

'Oh.' She smiled a fuzzy smile at me. 'Hullo.'

'Hullo, love.'

Waiting for the lift outside the Renal Unit, we debated whether or not to call it a day. Diana was dipping deep into her energy reserves – the formula went like this: one day out = two days in bed beforehand to prepare + three days afterwards to recover.

Was it worth pushing it to a week in bed merely for a couple of routine appointments?

We decided to debate the matter further over a Danish pastry at the WVS kiosk. The WVS tea was unpredictable and the coffee undrinkable, but the Danish pastries were a delight and Egon Ronay would have had an orgasm.

The lift arrived and, together with three other adults and a child in a pushchair, we squeezed ourselves into the tiny space. The adults behaved as adults always do in a lift. Two examined the ceiling for knotholes and the other stared over my left shoulder, fascinated by the control buttons. But children have no time for such nonsense. The pushchair and wheelchair faced one another – the occupants in an eyeball-to-eyeball confrontation, the child fascinated by the lady whose hands were strung together with plaster and struts.

'What's up with thee?'

'Gerald!' His mother rolled her eyes at the child and then returned them to the fascinating rivet in the lift wall.

'My hands don't work very well, so I'm having them mended.'

'Why are you in this?' He leaned forward and rattled the chair wheel.

'My legs don't work very well either.'

Gerald studied Diana's legs.

'They look all right.'

'Thank you, Gerald,' breathed Diana, fluttering her eyes at the boy.

The lift hummed to a halt and, as the doors opened, the sighs were audible.

Out in the wide corridor the pushchair took a slight lead, but gradually I drew the wheelchair level. Gerald whooped with delight.

'Let's have a race.'

'OK,' shouted Diana. 'Last one to the double doors is a cissy.'

Gerald braced himself to cope with the g forces, and then let out a cry of disappointment as his driver turned off down a branch line without a word.

The last we saw of Gerald he was peering over his shoulder, little face crumpled, eyes bright with indignation. Diana knew how he felt. In wheelchair as in pushchair, you are the helpless victim of the human engine.

'We could have beaten the kid,' muttered Diana.

'Left him standing,' I agreed. We reached the double doors.

'Where to? Hands, Plaster or Danish pastry?'

She considered these three pulsating options with a mounting excitement that bordered on near-hysteria.

'Let's go home,' she said. 'I'm knackered.'

4

'There are three pairs of pants missing,' Diana declared as we sorted out the washing on the bed.

After I had plucked all there was to pluck from the tumble dryer, I always humped it upstairs so that we could sort it out on the bed – it's called togetherness.

'You should have eight pairs, and there are only four here.'

'Then there are four pairs missing,' I pointed out.

'Three.'

'Four. We've found four and we should have eight – that's four.'

'Aren't you wearing any, then?'

One day I am going to learn to think before I open my mouth, but I have a feeling it's already too late.

I could hear the chink of Arthur Hind's milk crate as he rattled down the drive, and I went to meet him at the door. Arthur delivered real milk from real cows that had real names like Buttercup and Susie. I always suspected that, if Arthur was ever ill, Buttercup and Susie would bring it round instead.

'Morning, Deric. I wondered if you wanted any orange juice and are these yours?'

He was holding between forefinger and thumb a pair of Y-fronts that I had dropped on the drive after wrenching them from the tumble dryer in the cellar.

That gave me an idea. I pulled open the door of the washing machine to see if there was another pair of pants playing hide-and-seek. At first glance it was empty, but I was learning fast. I crouched down on my hands and knees so that I could see the roof of the machine and there, sucking in its cheeks and hanging on for grim life, was pair of pants number two – the cheeky ones with the flying hamster motif.

I couldn't find the third pair anywhere, but I knew that in a few weeks' time they would turn up, a good deal thinner and looking drawn and haggard, but otherwise none the worse for their experience.

For a couple of weeks I should have a full set, and then two more would make a break for it. I have never yet pulled from a washing machine all that I stuffed into it an hour earlier. I once lost a single-sized Paddington Bear duvet cover and a matching fitted sheet. I'm quite proud of that – it stands as my British national and all-comers' record.

I was halfway across the hall when the phone rang, and I picked up the receiver midway through the first ding. It was my mother.

'Deric – I wonder if you would do me a favour?'

Diana's voice floated down the stairs – she hadn't heard the phone.

'There's a pair of brown socks missing.'

I shouted back. 'I can't talk now, I'm on the phone.'

'I'm ever so sorry,' apologized my mother. 'I didn't realize.' And with that she put the phone down.

I rang her straight back.

'That was quick,' she said. 'I wonder if you could do me a favour?'

'Anything, love.' My mother is delightful, eccentric and seventy-two. The older she gets, the more delightful and eccentric she becomes.

'I wondered if you were going past my doctor's today?'

I never went past her doctor's – it was in Chesterfield, a twenty-five-mile round trip for me – but she never liked to feel she was putting me out.

'Yes, of course,' I said.

'Good.' She was pleased. 'Would you mind picking up my repeat prescription and, whilst you're there, would you pick up Nellie Elliot's as well?'

I never did find out what it was that Nellie Elliot suffered from, but my mother always said that she was a martyr to it.

Later that morning Rosie Cuff arrived to keep Diana company, and I had a chance to nip over to Chesterfield. Rosie and Keith were wonderful friends and nothing was too much trouble for them – so much so that I had to be careful when I asked a favour.

45

'Are you busy today, Rosie?'

'No.'

'Are you sure?'

'No – in fact I was thinking of popping round, if that's all right?'

'That would be terrific – I need to go out for an hour or two.'

'I'll be there in ten minutes.'

Rosie would let Keith break the news to their son Robert that the day trip to Harrogate was off, and she would be letting herself in at the back door in eight minutes flat. I had to be careful. Today, however, it was official – it had been arranged in advance, and so I kissed them both goodbye and drove over to Chesterfield.

After a morning in the factory I had laid up and cut fifty dozen split-front waist slips, survived an argument about the Christmas holidays and attempted to give the kiss of life to a geriatric sewing machine.

'See you in the morning' I shouted as I left. The silence that followed me told me that they would believe it when they saw it.

I called at the surgery, picked up my mother's prescription and made my way to the chemist's. I had to park a good quarter of a mile away and it was raining gently. The dispensary was crowded, but eventually a girl in a white coat took the prescription from me and I settled down for a long wait. I

46

was amusing myself trying to figure out whether I had normal, greasy or fly-away hair when the chemist himself appeared and bellowed: 'Mrs Longden.'

'Here,' I shouted, and all the customers giggled.

'Have you any idea what strength her sleeping tablets are?'

'I haven't,' I told him, and he sighed.

'I've tried ringing the surgery but there's nobody there – let me give you a tip. Never have a haemorrhage between one o'clock and three around here or you'll bleed to death. Is she on the phone?'

I told him she was, and we walked together behind the counter. I dialled the number and then passed him the phone.

'Ah! Mrs Longden,' he said when she answered. 'Your husband has just brought in a prescription.'

'Has he?' said my mother, sounding somewhat surprised.

'I'm her son,' I told him.

'Oh – I'm sorry, it's your son.'

'I didn't think it would be my husband,' said my mother. 'He's been dead fourteen years.'

'Well now, what it is, Mrs Longden,' began the chemist. 'Have you any idea what strength your sleeping tablets are?'

'I haven't,' said my mother.

'Have you still got the old bottle?'

'I'm afraid not.'

'Well, I'm awfully sorry, Mrs Longden – but

47

unless I know the strength I can't let you have any tablets for the time being.'

'Oh, that's all right,' said my mother happily. 'I don't take them myself – I never have. I don't believe in them.'

It took about thirty seconds for the chemist to run this information around his brain, and then he pulled himself together. He plucked the repeat prescription from my hand.

'But according to my records, Mrs Longden, you've been having sixty tablets a month for the past five years.'

'That's right,' my mother agreed. 'Nellie Elliot has most of them, and Gladys and Sarah have the odd one, and Mrs Cartwright from next door comes round if her sister's had a bad night the night before.'

The chemist looked at me with double-glazed eyes.

'Look, Mrs Longden. I'm not going to be able to let you have any sleeping tablets, and I'm going to ask your son to have a word with your doctor.'

'I quite understand,' said my mother – she's a good loser. 'Could you just put a few in a bottle for Nellie – only her doctor won't let her have any for herself.'

About an hour later I was standing at her door bearing Nellie's collection of bottles in a carrier bag, but only the blood pressure pills for my mother.

'I'm sorry about the sleeping tablets.'

'It's not me,' said my mother. 'It's Nellie I feel sorry for – especially after what she did for me.'

'What did Nellie do for you?' I wanted to know.

'Well, the other day she went into town and while she was there she popped into Woolworth's, and while she was in Woolworth's she went into that little booth to have her picture took for her bus pass. And when they came out there was four of them – so she's given me one for my bus pass.'

I sat on the settee staring at my mother's bus pass, and staring back at me, set in Harris tweed shoulders, was the crimplene face of Nellie Elliot.

'What does the bus conductor say?' I asked.

'He always says I should sue Woolworth's – but I think it's good of Nellie, don't you?'

She studied the photograph and I couldn't help thinking that perhaps it was a good job Nellie had had it taken before she came cold turkey off the sleeping tablets. God knows what she would look like in a month's time.

'Would you like a cup of coffee?' My mother began to heave herself out of the low armchair.

'I'd love a cup, please.'

'Are you sure – I'm having one.'

'All right, I will then – if you're having one.'

'It's no trouble.'

'Well, if it's no trouble, I'd love a cup. Thank you.'

I followed her into the kitchen.

49

'Don't look at the cat – he gets embarrassed when he's thrutching.'

I looked at the cat and caught him in mid-thrutch. Whisky was grinning at me from the cat litter tray, and with his eyes half closed in concentration he was the spitting image of Malcolm Muggeridge. He was a funny-looking cat. He was black and white, but not as daintily marked as other cats. He was black down the left side and white down the right. When you looked at him head on, he seemed to be two cats leaning against each other.

'How is Diana?'

'Not so bad at the moment – she has to go down to London again soon for tests.'

'Poor girl – she's lovely. Are you sure you won't have a coffee?'

'Go on, then.'

She reached for another mug with a sigh.

'I wish you would make your mind up.'

Whisky lifted himself an inch or two above the cat litter and peered around for tell-tale signs of success. There weren't any, but he shuffled the sawdust just in case and then strolled over to his saucer of cod in butter sauce.

This would be about his second year on cod in butter sauce. Before that he had had a three-year stretch on rabbit. If my mother discovered you liked something, she kept it coming. I had gone straight from being breast-fed on to egg and chips, and I stayed on them until I joined the Air Force.

My mother also cast a weather eye over the cat litter and then, plucking a packet of bran flakes from the shelf, she scattered a goodly portion over the cod in butter sauce and approximately twice as much over the cat's head.

'He needs the roughage,' she said knowingly, but Whisky shook himself vigorously, gave a disgusted look at his ruined lunch and, picking up his pipe cleaner, strolled off into the drawing room. He never went anywhere without his pipe cleaner. He walked about the house with it stuck in his mouth at a jaunty angle, looking for all the world like a Somerset yokel complete with straw.

'Come on,' said my mother, gathering up the two mugs of coffee, and we went to join Whisky. 'I want to phone Ruby Blackmore in Whetstone and I can't find her number,' she complained. 'Wouldn't you think the telephone people would be able to help? All they would have to do would be to set a girl up in a room with all the telephone directories and then we could ring her and she could tell us the number.'

'You can,' I told her. 'It's called Directory Enquiries – you just dial 192.'

She considered my information as she picked bran flakes from Whisky's head.

'They never do anything until you complain, do they? Give 'em a ring for me.'

'No, you do it,' I said, pulling the phone over. 'Then you'll be able to do it again. Just dial 192.'

She dialled carefully, with notebook and pencil at the ready.

'What town?' demanded a voice.

'Er . . . Chesterfield.'

'Name?'

'Longden.'

'Initial?'

'A.M.'

'Address?'

'147 Old Road.'

'The number is 274931.'

'274 . . .?' My mother wrote carefully.

. . .931.'

'Thank you.' She finished jotting down the number and then, glancing a couple of times from her notebook to the telephone, she exclaimed: 'Bloody hell – she's spot on.'

I looked at Whisky and Whisky, his back leg high round his earhole, looked at me.

'But you didn't want *your* number – you wanted Ruby's.'

'I know.' She nudged Whisky with her foot and he fell over. 'But she didn't ask the right questions.'

I persuaded Directory Enquiries to part with Ruby's number, and then dialled Diana.

'Tell Rosie it's all right to leave me on my own,' she ordered. 'She's got a meal to get ready.'

'Only if you'll promise to stay in bed until I get home.'

'I promise.'

'Swear on the Bible.'

'I haven't got a Bible handy. I've got a *Woman's Own* – will that do?'

'Place your hand on Virginia Ironside and say after me: " I swear that I will stay in bed."'

'I swear that I will stay in bed.'

'So help me God.'

'You silly sod.'

'YOU CAN GO HOME, ROSIE,' I yelled.

I knew Diana only too well. As soon as she was on her own, she liked to explore. By hanging on to the furniture she could negotiate her way around the bedroom and move all the ornaments an inch to the left, where God had intended them to be. She could straighten duvets and square off towels and remove thumbprints from mirrors with her dressing gown elbow. Since she couldn't protect herself with her hands if she fell, she had collected black eyes, bruises and broken bones. But the danger area lay at the top of the stairs. There she had nothing to hold on to, and twice already she had performed her famous double somersault with triple flip from top to bottom. As I turned the key and pushed open the kitchen door I heard her voice.

'Don't worry – I'm all right.'

I raced through the hall to the stairs. She was jammed on her back halfway down – her feet hooked around the newel post and her head hard against the wall. Her nose was bloodied and her eyes were rolling pinpricks.

'I slipped.'

I kissed her and tried to lift her. I've always admired those Mills & Boon heroes who sweep the heroine into their arms and race off up the cliff to lay her down beneath the jacaranda trees.

I had to get Diana back in bed. Christ! – if I dropped her.

She smiled a drunken smile. 'I slipped.'

She would have to go to hospital, so perhaps it would be better to take her downstairs. Doing my best not to hurt her, I half carried and half hauled her across the hall and laid her down on the settee. At the window I could see a window cleaner hanging at right-angles from his ladder and doing his best not to see what we were up to. He whistled 'Just one cornetto' and his hat dropped off.

Diana, grey and shaking now, smiled thinly.

'I know – you slipped. Don't worry, I'll look after you,' I said, and then I chased upstairs to the bathroom.

I grabbed a thick dressing gown and a blanket, and then as I turned I saw them, hanging from a line over the bathtub. There – tallest on the left, shortest on the right – dripping down into the bath from the line were the large teddy bear, the small teddy bear and the cuddly kangaroo complete with sodden baby staring miserably from her pouch. The purple rabbit looked thoroughly depressed, as did the bright yellow chicken – Snoopy, however, looked wonderfully white and both he and Woodstock grinned happily as they dangled in mid-air. At least Diana had another job she could cross from her list on the bedside table – I had wondered for some weeks what 'Scrub chicken' meant, but I couldn't ask her as I wasn't supposed to know the list was there.

I pushed open the front door and lifted Diana from the settee. Down a couple of steps and I was on the drive and heading towards the car at the top, carrying a blanket with a face peeping out.

The window cleaner shouted 'Good evening' at my back as I struggled with the car door. I hooked one finger in the lock and opened the door an inch, then, resting Diana on my knees, tucked my toe round the door edge and fell backwards on my bottom on the pavement.

'Could you give me a hand?'

He was by my side in an instant – chivalrous deeds performed by request only – and he held the door as I lifted Diana into the car. He bent towards her to offer words of comfort.

'I've had to put it up – it's two pounds fifty now.'

Diana smiled, her eyes examining the inside of her head. 'I slipped.'

He hesitated, plucking up courage for what he was about to say. 'But . . . you can pay next time.'

'Thank you,' I shouted as I slammed the car door, and he turned and walked sadly back to his ladder and picked his leather up off the lawn.

5

The Casualty ward at the Chesterfield Royal is a series of curtained stalls behind which doctors and nurses perform major and minor miracles. Along the wall facing the stalls are a row of stacking chairs which seat a collection of anxious minders – parents, wives, husbands, lovers, friends and enemies. Behind one curtain an old lady tries hard not to cry out as a kidney stone works its wicked way through her system. Behind another, a six-foot rugby player threatens to swing for anyone who tries to give him an anti-tetanus jab.

'All right,' says the doctor, 'but don't come back here when your leg drops off.'

A drunk staggers up and down the lines of chairs, playing to the audience.

'I am perfectly crappable – they say I am incrappable, but I am perfectly crappable.'

'Sit down,' orders a civilian receptionist from behind a small desk at the far end of the room.

'Mary!' The drunk seems to know her. 'My lovely Mary from the Hope and Anchor.'

She blushes and busies herself with paperwork until a nurse shouts.

'Mary – can you spare a moment?'

He did know her! – and the audience buzzes, but then they fall silent as a leather-lunged nurse, from behind a curtain, poses the question, 'When did you last have your bowels open?'

The audience wait with ears cocked for the answer. A timid, very private voice answers.

'It must be all of three weeks.'

Twenty faces wince in unison at the information and then, having filed it away, they turn their attention back to the drunk.

He is sitting on Mary's desk awaiting her return, and to kill time he sings snatches from *The Chocolate Soldier*.

Diana was in the end stall, and had been for the best part of an hour. A young nurse had conducted a superficial investigation that amounted to a limb count and Mary had taken her name, rank and serial number, and, so far, that was that.

Then a young doctor appeared from the service alley at the back of the stalls. He took my place on the edge of the bed and gently stroked Diana's forehead where a blue-black bruise was oozing to the surface. He shone a light in her eyes and then asked: 'Can you touch my nose?'

Diana focused, then took aim and with a crisp, neat jab poked him straight in the eye with the wire strut of Fred's left hand. He blinked bravely at first and then mopped up the tears with the corner of a sheet. I knew how he felt – it often happened to me when Diana turned over in the night, and it hurt.

'Can you touch your own nose?'

Diana grinned her 'Course I can' grin and, taking aim like a drunken darts player, jabbed herself in the eye, this time with the plaster thumb extension.

I borrowed the corner of the sheet from the doctor and dried her tears.

'I think we'll keep her in,' he declared, standing up. 'I'll go and make the arrangements.'

Diana smiled at the nurse who was no longer there, and then she turned to me.

'Did I do all right?'

'You did fine.'

The smile was replaced by a naïve, somewhat puzzled, faraway look that often took over when the pain was at its worst. It seemed to ask so many questions and it always turned my heart over.

'I think I'll go to sleep now.'

'All right, darling – I'll be here.'

She closed her eyes and fell asleep instantly. I stroked her arm and for some minutes listened to the sounds around me . . . .

'Can you remember how many pills you took? Come on, talk to me – how many were there in this bottle?' . . .

'How did he come to swallow a ball bearing?'

'I bought him a bagatelle set – it were on top of wardrobe for Christmas. He found it – he pulled pinger and ball shot down his throat.' . . .

58

'Did the son take her out in a wheelchair?'

'I think so.'

'Did he or didn't he?'

'I think so.'

'Bloody hell! Sister! They've pinched another wheelchair.' . . .

Suddenly the doctor reappeared in the stall.

'By the way – don't let her fall asleep, will you?'

I tried to wake her, whispering at first and then louder, but she might have been hibernating for all the effect it had. I couldn't shake her because of the hurt, and so I slipped my hand under the sheet and stroked her in a secret place, the location of which wild horses wouldn't drag from me.

Her reaction was a slow smile and then a line straight out of a 'B' movie.

'Where am I?'

'You're in hospital, love.'

She tried to curl herself up into a ball.

'Oh, no. Not again.'

Nick had put together a supper for us and as we ate I filled him in on the events of the day. From the age of three onwards he has always given me good advice.

'Now – we must think positively.'

'Of course.'

'Mum might be in hospital for a few days.'

'Right.'

'So you have a chance to do some work without any interruption.'

59

'Yes – except for visiting . . . .'

'I'll visit in the afternoon – that will leave you free during the day. You can fit in the trips to London and Manchester and visit in the evenings.'

'Right.'

'I'll organize the factory – which is the most important order?'

'Henry Margolis.'

'I'll ring Henry – what have you got to do for tomorrow?'

'Write a piece for Radio Derby. A sports review for Radio Nottingham and record that piece about spiders for "Woman's Hour". Then there's the column for the paper, Ian Gregory wants it by lunchtime and . . . .'

'Right. Off you go upstairs then and get cracking – I'll bring your coffee up there.'

I stood up. 'What about your job?' He was doing well at the *Derbyshire Times* and I didn't want to cause him any problems.

'I'll handle that – off you go.'

Nick began to clear the table. I paused at the door.

'I think I'd like to see your mum in the afternoon – just tomorrow.'

'No. I'll go in the afternoon – you go at night. Mum would agree.'

He balanced the plates on one hand and headed for the kitchen. I headed for the office.

He had always had this air of authority – he had hit maturity at the age of three and he had approached any crisis since with a clean, crisp mind and a grasp of the essentials that was to be genuinely admired. Added to that he was loving, generous to a fault and loyal beyond question. Pity he was too big to clip round the earhole.

My mother and I arrived at the hospital five minutes before opening time. I wanted to be alone with Diana, but for the first time in a long time she was in a hospital close enough for my mother to visit, and she was determined to see that her daughter-in-law was being looked after properly. As we walked in through the main door a rather distinguished-looking man held it open for us – he carried a black bag with a stethoscope tucked under the handle. He would be in his early sixties, with immaculate grey hair curling over his collar, and he wore a dark suit and a homburg. Central casting had obviously sent him to play the part of the leading neurosurgeon.

He smiled in recognition. 'Hullo, Mrs Longden.'

'Hullo, Raymond,' said my mother, and swept past him into the hall.

'Who was that?' I wanted to know.

'That's Bessie Rimmington's eldest lad – he used to deliver our meat.'

'Did he?' I looked back at the retreating figure – all proudly pin-striped and Asprey-tiepinned.

'He was always falling off his bike,' said my mother. 'He was all right whilst his basket was full, but when it was empty he used to fall over backwards. He never did get the hang of it – I think he was a bit peculiar.'

'He seems to have done all right for himself since then.' It seemed only fair to put in a good word for him. 'I think he's a doctor.'

'Well, he'd never have made a butcher.'

My mother isn't easily impressed.

'Which ward is she in?'

'Margaret Greave,' I told her. 'It's this . . .'

'I know which way it is – it's quicker through here.'

She spun me around and we took a short cut through an alley of tiny cubicles in which patients seemed to be either whipping on nighties or whipping them off. I tried to look straight ahead.

In no time at all we were outside the ward. A small knot of visitors huddled together in the corridor, Lucozade and daffodils at the ready, waiting for the word from the sister that they could go in. It isn't that my mother is rude – she just doesn't understand that there is such a thing as a pecking order. She threaded her way through the throng and pushed open the glass doors. The sister came over to bar her path.

'I'm afraid the doctor is still doing his rounds,' she explained.

'That's all right,' smiled my mother. 'He won't bother me.' And she weaved her way up the ward, peering closely at the occupant of each bed, looking for Diana.

62

The third bed up on the right was surrounded by a curtain. My mother put her eye to a chink and then turned and smiled delightedly to where I was still standing cowardly with the crowd.

'It's Lily Goodhind as was,' she announced, and then disappeared in through the curtain.

The sister followed her through the gap, closing it behind her, and we all stood in silence, daffodils frozen in salute, waiting for the next scene to unfold.

Minutes passed and then the sister emerged. She pulled back the curtain and made a door-sized opening. Through it emerged first the consultant, immediately followed by a houseman and a physio-therapist and then, in duckling style, three student doctors, Florence Nightingale and two Chinese nurses. The sister completed the drawing of the curtain to reveal my mother, sitting on a chair at the bedside, her face a mask of concentration, chatting to 'Lily Goodhind as was'. There was a spontaneous burst of applause from behind the glass doors, at which the sister decided to let the peasants in as well, and as I drew level with the third bed on the right I nodded to my mother. She nodded back.

'That's mine,' she said to Lily, 'but he's got a lovely wife.'

Diana lay back on her pillows and smiled. The bruise on her forehead had crept around her eye and raked her cheek.

'How are you, darling?'

'I'm fine.'

I funnelled the spare nightdress into her locker and arranged the tangerines alongside Nick's grapes.

'How are you really?'

'Bloody awful.'

There was something strange about her head movements. I couldn't work it out straightaway, and then I realized that, instead of swivelling her eyes, she was moving her whole head – her eyes remaining set in their sockets.

'Have you got a migraine?'

'No – it's my eyes, they're heavy like marbles. I can feel them all the time. When I move them – they grind. It's as though . . . as though they need oiling.'

I became conscious of my own eyes – of every transient flit and flicker. They never stopped moving. A couple of seconds ago I hadn't been aware of my eyes – they were just for seeing with.

'I want to come home. They're too interested in me here.'

Every time she went into a fresh hospital it was the same. She represented a challenge and eager minds wanted to prod and probe. Then as test after painful test showed absolutely nothing she was shuffled off into a backwater, eventually to be discharged in an embarrassed silence.

'I won't let them. You're due down in the Maudsley soon. They'll sort something out this time.'

The marble eyes swung round on me. The mouth

64

said nothing but the eyes told me not to be so daft. Mr Polkey at the Maudsley was one of the finest neurologists in the world and he had never let Diana down, but he had made it clear that he had exhausted just about every possibility. He was to have one more stab at it.

Diana was tiring fast, so I talked and she pretended to listen. I wanted to have a word with the doctors but that had to be done during the daytime. Tomorrow I would visit with Nick – he could occupy Diana whilst I prowled around for information.

I saw my mother rise to her feet as she bade goodbye to Lily. She stared up the ward and began to thread her drunken way towards us. She could see the beds but she had no idea who was lying in them until she was within about three feet of her victim, and so she swayed from this side of the ward to that – peering as though through a fog at each and every occupant. The conversation at the bedside would stop as my mother approached to examine the body – then it would start up again, nervously, as she drew away. Eventually she recognized my outline at the side of Diana's bed and she waved vigorously in our general direction.

'Hello, love,' she shouted to Diana.

'Hello, Annie,' exclaimed the old lady in the next bed. She was sitting up, swathed in brushed nylon, and knitting what appeared to be a huge Brillo pad.

She had a lovely, lived-in face and her wrinkles seemed to have been picked out with eyeliner.

'Minnie Bonsall!' cried my mother in recognition. 'It must be fifteen years.'

'Eighteen,' declared Minnie. 'Arthur's been dead eighteen years this week – it was at the funeral.'

'That's right.' My mother pulled up a chair and tucked herself in beside Minnie's bed.

'How is Arthur?'

'He's dead.'

'Oh aye, of course. Shouldn't you be in Bournemouth?'

'It was full of old folk,' Minnie confided. 'I couldn't stand it any longer.'

Diana and I talked for another ten minutes or so and then the sister entered briskly carrying a large bell. She rang it at the far end of the ward and she rang it in the middle. Then she rang it in my mother's left ear, which was a mistake – it's her deaf side. I began to put together the bits and pieces that Diana wanted me to recycle at home, and then my mother appeared at my elbow.

'Minnie Bonsall's knitting a dishcloth.' So that's what it was. She sat down and took Diana's hand.

'How are you, love?'

'I'm fine. Thank you for coming.'

'Don't be silly – you need company when you're not well. I brought you some orange juice, but I've given it to Minnie Bonsall.'

★

I drew up outside my mother's house and switched the engine off. She was on a high after seeing so many old faces, and she was still chattering to me as I walked round the car to help her out. Hauling my mother out of the car was never an easy task. She could have studied the Queen Mother for a month without getting the hang of it. She would have tackled an exit from the Irish State Coach just as she tackled the Citroën. As I opened the passenger door to help her out, she spun herself round on her bottom so that her legs were pointing towards the door, then she lowered her body gently across both the front seats – the steering wheel an inch or so above her nose. Now horizontal, she inched her way towards me – her skirt creeping up towards her neck. First a glimpse of underskirt, then a vast expanse of American tan tights and then, finally, a panoramic sweep of Spirella corsetry as she swung herself to her feet.

'They do make 'em awkward to get out of, don't they?'

Once, during a similar performance outside Chesterfield Town Hall, a young man had advanced from the sizeable crowd who were watching and asked: 'Can I be of any help? I'm a male nurse.'

It was some time before I could convince him that here was a very fit and robust old lady who simply had her own way of doing things. Usually I rejoiced in her eccentricity. She has never embarrassed me – only delighted me – but today I was a little disenchanted with her.

Never once on the journey home had she mentioned Diana. I had listened to her account of Lily Goodhind's kidneys and Minnie Bonsall's bowels with mounting impatience. But she seemed to have completely forgotten her three-minute vigil at Diana's bedside.

I opened the front gate and saw her down the path. At the door she turned to kiss me good night.

'Keep an eye on that girl. Did you see her eyes? There's something wrong with those eyes – I wouldn't be surprised if that fall hasn't done more damage than they think, and her voice was just like it is on the phone before she has one of her really bad spells. I can always tell – she was sitting up peculiar. I think she ought to be in Sheffield where they know more about her.'

I kissed her again and then once more for good measure. She smiled shyly – she doesn't like you to overdo it.

On the way home I stopped off at the factory to sort out this and that, and then at the White Hart at Walton for a whisky and water with a man who told me more about his piles than I ever wished to know.

Nick was waiting for me as I tucked the car away in the garage. He took a sip of tea from a Snoopy mug and said, 'The hospital have just been on the phone. Mum's had a relapse – they're very worried about her, she's in a lot of pain, so they've sent her over to Sheffield. They said that they would know more about her case at the Hallamshire. We'll go in my car.'

I took Snoopy from him and finished off his tea, and by half past midnight we were walking through yet another Casualty ward. This time the drunk would have been in good company. They were spilling out of the cubicles, and a dozen or so had been laid out to dry on mattresses along the corridor. In a few hours they would hose down the floors ready for a fresh start.

A nurse picked her way through the stupefied debris as she escorted us to the main hospital.

'Bloody weekend again,' she said.

6

Sheffield's Royal Hallamshire Hospital is an enormous, purpose-built Portakabin of a building with all the charm and character of an international airport. The revolutionary heating system bakes patients and nurses alike at gas mark six on some days and forces them into thermal vests on others, when only patients with temperatures in the high one hundred and twenties rest easy in their beds.

The nurse who had escorted us from Casualty left us outnumbered by a bank of lifts in the foyer and returned to her drunks and would-be suicides. The large hall was empty, but I still had time to work my way through 'It Pays to Enrich Your Word Power', 'My Most Unforgettable Character', and 'Humour in Uniform' before the welcome 'ding' of a lift broke through the silence. Nick had eschewed the *Reader's Digest* in favour of the *People's Friend*, and he stowed it away inside his jacket in order to discover the Laird's dark secret in his own sweet time.

The wards were tucked away behind two sets of double doors which opened on to a brightly lit corridor. Midway along was the nurses' station and opposite that a series of bays, each containing four to six beds. The quiet was punctuated by the heavy breathing of the Mogadon set, rough sandpaper snores and the odd mattress-muffled breaking of wind. The nurse was extremely young and incredibly beautiful and Nick was pleased that he had hidden the *People's Friend* well away out of sight. She led us down the corridor and into one of the bays.

'Mrs Longden was very poorly when she was admitted. Her vision was affected and she complained of head pains.'

'Did a doctor look at her?'

'The consultant is coming in the morning. The duty doctor gave her an injection and she's asleep now – she's very comfortable.'

Most of us are comfortable when we are unconscious.

'Did the doctor say what he thought might be happening?'

'He thought it might be just concussion – but then he saw her notes . . . .' She broke off.

Diana was sleeping peacefully as Nick and I pulled up chairs either side of the bed. Her hair was wild and spread over the pillow. She wore no make-up and I took hold of her hand as it lay on the cover. Three fingernails were immaculately varnished – the other two were pearly white. She must have been halfway through painting them just before she fell down the stairs.

It took Diana a whole day to paint her nails. She would set out her stall on the bedside table – cotton wool, remover and varnish. I would loosen the bottle tops and then she would start. With the cotton wool held between first and second fingers she would work away at the old varnish, rubbing the finger against the wool rather than the other way around. Two fingernails would be wiped clean and then it was time for a rest. I would be called in on occasions to hold back the skin at the side of the nails so that she could work at the awkward bits, but on no account was I allowed to either wipe or paint. This was her mountain and she would climb it without ropes.

The morning would be taken up with the cleaning and then, in the afternoon – the artistic bit. The brush would swing loosely between the fingers, held high up towards the web. Gently she would draw it the length of the nail and then, revolving the finger slightly, retrace her steps. One finger and then a rest. Two more fingers and then a sleep. I would be called upon to massage her arms, and then the assault on the second hand would begin. As her eyes grew tired she would hold them wide and unblinking so as to focus, and as her hands became unbearably weary she would smudge the nails and daub her fingers. Then out would come the cotton wool again until, as the evening closed in, ten impeccable little fingernails would be laid out to dry, blood red against the white sheets.

It was my job to clean the nail varnish from sheets, nightdress and Fred's hands, and after that was done I would lie beside her on the bed and we would watch Jim Rockford limp his way around Los Angeles. During the dull bits she would stare at her hands with quiet pride and then hold them up for me to admire.

'They look great – you've done a good job.'

Just before we switched out the lights to sleep she would allow me one more private view and then, after a kiss, I would wait for her to say:

'I'm not sure I like this colour – I think I'll lighten it tomorrow.' She was a very easy woman to love.

It was now two-thirty in the morning and Nick looked weary. Our conversation, which normally flowed easily, was forced and artificial.

'You OK?'

'Yes – fine.'

'You don't have to stay.'

'No – I want to.'

A hospital ward in the early hours of the morning, with bodies groaning in the half light, inhibits social behaviour every bit as much as does a VD clinic at lunchtime. Diana didn't need us right now, so why were we hanging on? We both loved her – we had nothing to prove. Perhaps, as much as wanting to do the right thing, it was wanting to be seen to do the right thing. We were achieving nothing – but we each didn't want the other, or the nurse for that matter, to think we didn't care.

And in the morning we could say to Diana; 'We sat by the bed all night.'

'You shouldn't have.'

'Don't be silly.' . . .

The nurse arrived with three cups of tea and perched on the edge of the bed. I followed Nick's gaze – she really did have great ankles. We talked in fits and starts, all of us looking at Diana as though not wanting to cut her out of the conversation.

'Why don't you both go home? There's really nothing you can do tonight.'

'If she wakes?'

'She won't – not tonight. I'll tell her you were here in the morning.'

We finished our tea and bent in turn to kiss Diana. The decision had been made for us and the responsibility lifted from our shoulders. We said good night to the nurse and walked out into the twilight.

Guilt can make pillocks of us all.

A few hours later I woke my half-doped son. With a beatific smile on his face and with padded headphones strapped to either side of his head, he looked like a half-baked rabbit. As I tapped him on the shoulder his left hand searched for his duvet. The duvet had a life of its own and roamed about the bedroom at will. Sometimes it was on top of the wardrobe – mostly it was on the floor. As I watched, it crawled across the bedside table on its way to having a good scratch on the bookshelf.

Every morning Nick would wake early, slip on his headphones and flick on a pre-selected disc. This was supposed to ease him gently into the day so that he wouldn't tremble at breakfast, and every morning he would sleep through one side of a long-playing record. I slipped the headphones from his ears and the whole room was filled with the sophisticated sounds of Wreckless Eric. I hadn't heard Wreckless Eric for years – Nick must have been in a nostalgic mood last night.

I switched off the music and the disc ground to a painful halt. The quiet almost hurt, and gradually the furniture settled down and the floorboards stopped dancing and went back to their seats. All I could hear was the sound of Nick's gentle snoring and a rustle down in the kitchen as the duvet opened a second packet of cornflakes.

When Sally lived at home the situation was critical. Her bedroom was on the other side of us and Diana and I lived in a musical San Andreas Fault, with Kate Bush's Heights a'Wuthering in one ear whilst Max Boyce assaulted the other live from Pontypool. This stereo vault situation was due to be revived – I was to meet her off the train from Holland at lunchtime.

Without the music Nick would wake in a few minutes. If I needed to rouse him instantly, I merely had to whisper in his ear: 'Your car's on fire – I think it's electrical.' This had been known to have him standing naked in the drive with the bonnet up in thirty-five seconds flat.

The train was three hotdogs, a packet of Maltesers and five coffees late, and the day was very cold. The only entertainment came in the shape of a large black lady who swept the buffet with a broom and a smile and sang gospel songs at people eating cheese sandwiches. Her only opposition had been moved on by the police during his twenty-third rendition of 'Oh, Mein Papa', and she took over centre stage like a natural.

'Is your train late, honey?'

'Yes.'

'Never mind, honey – as long as you got Jesus.'

'I've got Jesus, love – it's my daughter I'm worried about.'

'What's she look like?'

'Well she's got . . .' I had no idea what colour her hair was. It was black when she had left, but it changed colour with the seasons – it could be red now that it was autumn. 'It's been a long time.'

'Never mind. My husband left me twelve years ago but the Good Lord will bring him back – and when he does I'm going to beat the shit out of him.'

She glided down the buffet on her broom singing, 'What a friend we have in Jesus', and bent to cheer up an accountant.

I've seen her on practically every main line station in the country sweeping out the buffets. I believe she spends most of her time at St Pancras and Euston, but obviously British Rail like her to tour now and then.

When Sally arrived I recognized her immediately – she was the most beautiful woman on the train. She wore a chunky roll-neck sweater that wrapped neatly around her bottom, and a pair of my thermal long johns tucked into high black boots; her purple-black hair fell about her shoulders and she was totally unaware that three young men chewing McEwan's lager cans were examining her backside at close quarters. As I hugged her, they moved on with a muted whistle and a hiss of disappointment. I felt old enough to be her father.

She looked around. 'Mum not here?'

'She couldn't make it, love – too cold.'

'She's all right?'

'Yes, fine – let's go and have a coffee – I have a friend who runs the buffet.'

Holland was to have been a new start for Sally, but it hadn't quite worked out.

A ballet dancer from the age of three, she realized ten years later that she wasn't going to make it in one of the big companies and so eventually she qualified as a teacher and began to torture little girls in Matlock. The trouble was that the only men she met were aged around seven years old and had an overwhelming desire to point their toes and wear tights.

The answer was to be a beauty therapist. 'You can work anywhere, Dad, in hotels and on the big liners – you meet very interesting people.' I suppose that's true and it did sound glamorous – but after studying at college for three years she discovered that even interesting people find it hard to make good conversation whilst having their bikini line waxed and superfluous hair removed from their top lip. Their eyes water a lot – but they say very little. As for working in exotic locations, her first job, after some local experience, was in a small salon in Putney – a place not noted for either its hotels or its passing liners.

It was in *The Lady* that she spotted the advert for a nanny 'with a diplomatic family in The Hague'.

Some misguided friends tried to talk her out of the idea.

'Do you think you ought to leave your mother when she's so ill?'

'Your place is with her really, isn't it?'

'I can see the strain in your dad's face.'

As though the thought had never occurred to her. Diana and I had been working on her guilt for some time. Before Diana became ill we had been closely connected with a disabled club and we had seen many twenty-year-old daughters who stayed at home to look after mother – many were still at it in their mid-forties.

A week before she was due to leave she sat on Diana's bed and said, 'I've made my mind up – I'm not leaving you.'

'Fine,' Diana had said. 'You can stay as long as you like, but everything you possess will be out on the drive on the 14th.'

Sally loved Holland but, although the English family were very decent to her, they were rather formal and she found the life restrictive and unfulfilling. She stuck it for just over a year and left on good terms. She had applied for jobs back in the beauty business, and in a fortnight would be butchering top lips once more, this time in exotic Leicester.

The Hallamshire was filling up with visitors. The WVS ladies in the snack bar were instructing a new recruit in tea-urn technology, and a long queue waited without complaint and studied Sally's longjohns with some interest as she bought a bunch of flowers from the stall opposite.

I'd bought the pants to counter the biting cold of the press box during football commentaries. I could never understand why all my leather-jacketed colleagues seemed as warm as toast, whilst I shivered under two anoraks. Then I discovered Damart, and my Saturday afternoons became bearable. I'd sent them to Sally after I discovered, in a Liverpool toilet, that I had bought large ladies' instead of medium men's, and that there was no little flap at the front. I'd lived in mortal fear of being hit by a truck, and here was Sally sporting them in public – but then she didn't have my knees.

We worked our way up to ward E2, where Diana was sitting up in bed supported by pillows. From her head sprouted a mass of wires connected to a sort of portable radio thing fastened by a belt to her waist. Sally fell upon her and I ate a couple of tangerines at the foot of the bed whilst they hugged and kissed and talked all at the same time. By the time they had run out of steam, a nurse had told me that the portable radio was in fact a twenty-four-hour electro-encephalograph to measure her brain waves.

'They're measuring my brain waves,' said Diana proudly. 'They're hoping that I'll have a blackout so they can measure that.'

I was pleased that I had been able to produce Sally out of the hat and that the doctors had got cracking with the EEG. Usually the first two days in hospital seemed to be packed with inactivity and I could predict the pattern of Diana's mood – we'd been through it all so many times.

On the first day one of the doctors would be quite dishy, but all the others would be idiots and the nurses couldn't give a toss. That is except the one who remembered Diana from her last visit and who came in to see her even though it was her day off. And the food would be lousy. By the second day all the doctors would be terrific except the dishy one who would turn out to be a self-centred prat – the nurses would be fantastic bar none and the little fat one, whom Diana didn't like at first, would be a bundle of fun. Only one impression would remain constant – the food was always lousy. It was a sort of institutionalization process that she had to go through before she settled.

As Diana's initial burst of energy ran out Sally took over the conversation, whilst I ate more tangerines and kept a watch on Diana's eyes for tell-tale signs of exhaustion. Before too long it became clear that she was near the end of her tether and I stepped in.

'Is there anything you want me to bring in tonight?'

As she dictated I made a list on the back of an envelope. Goods to be ferried into hospital on one side, and little jobs for me to do on the other.

Whenever anyone dictates to me I write as fast as I can so as not to keep them waiting. I don't want their train of thought to be interrupted by any hesitation on my part. So I write very quickly with an uncharacteristic flourish, giving extravagant tails to my Ys and curly tops to my Ts, and I mutter MMM-MmmMUGH! after every item is duly written down – and then I stab a big dot to indicate that I've got it. Anyone who dictates to me is always very impressed – especially by my MMMMmmMUGH! and the dot, which seems to emphasize my efficiency. Everyone is impressed, that is, except Diana. She knows that, within the hour, there will be at least five items that I shan't be able to decipher.

'Have you got all that?'

'MMMMmmMUGH!'

'Read it back to me.'

So I read it back, starting with the fresh orange juice and ending with the burgundy nightdress that I was to wash, but under no circumstances put through the tumble dryer.

'Have I said a box of tissues?' Diana asked craftily, spot checking a second time.

'MMMMmmMUGH!' I said, giving the tissues an extra dot.

There was little more she could do to ensure that I could read my own writing – but we both knew that I had picked up full marks simply because the list was fresh in my mind.

In a few hours I wouldn't be able to make head nor tail of at least three of the items – and that was on a good day.

At home Sally spent some time rearranging her bedroom, and I squatted beside her sorting out the washing and attempting to unravel my list. My writing really is appalling. The second item was 'Skidway Otter'. That's the best I could do, 'Skidway Otter' – two words.

I pushed the list over to Sally.

'What does that say?'

'Skidway Otter,' she declared proudly.

'Thank you.' I had hoped for more than that.

'Don't mention it,' she said, and then added, 'What is Skidway Otter?'

'I haven't the slightest idea,' I told her. 'Nor have I any idea what is a "Rumbling Stain" or "Garbage".'

'Garbage is what you throw out.'

'That's what your mother will do with me,' I told her, and began to sort the washing into two piles.

Sally took charge of the non-ironing pile.

'I haven't seen this before,' she said, holding up a shortie burgundy nightdress. 'It's the same style as her full-length one.'

'It *is* her full-length one.' I grabbed it miserably – half of it seemed to have disappeared in the tumble dryer.

No matter how hard I try, I have never really come to terms with the domestic side of life. I put on a good act, but I don't concentrate hard enough – my mind wanders and I finish up with only half a nightdress and a Skidway Otter.

That night at the hospital the sister beckoned to me as we passed her desk.

'You'll find Diana drugged up to the eyeballs tonight, I'm afraid – she had a blackout and fell out of bed.'

'Is she all right?'

'Yes. She suffered some bruising and quite a lot of pain, but she'll be all right. I believe she was showing the lady in the next bed how she could bend her thumb right backwards. Mrs Partridge is quite short-sighted and Diana tried to get too close – at least that's what Mrs Partridge says.'

It was Diana's party trick and quite horrific – it was a wonder Mrs Partridge hadn't had the blackout.

We hurried in to see Diana, and the nurse shouted: 'We got the blackout on the EEG – that was lucky.'

Diana was in a world of her own, smiling faintly – her hair was matted with the glue that had secured the wires, her forehead black with the old bruising, blue with the new. She would have hated it, but she knew nothing.

Sally and I held a hand each and sat silently. Other patients and visitors came over every now and then to sympathize. Apparently her fall had been spectacular – she had finished up trapped double under the bed and had to be removed by a two-nurse team.

It's strange – when someone you love is always ill, always in pain. It is impossible to sustain the hurt at a high level. You become used to witnessing pain and suffering – it's the norm, and the sadness is pitched to such a point over a long period that it is not possible to accommodate the peaks. The result is a continuing numbness that is set to a certain frequency, and the occasional crisis just bounces off.

We just sat and loved her and then, as the ward began to clear of visitors, she saw Sally as though for the first time and began to talk softly. I watched the two of them together, so much alike, and felt very lucky.

The nurses moved in, swishing curtains and

popping pills, making it clear that it was time for us to leave.

'I couldn't find a Skidway Otter,' I told Diana. 'And they were completely out of Rumbling Stains.'

'Doesn't matter,' smiled Diana dreamily. 'Try the Co-op – they're very good.'

She was fast asleep again before we left.

'Well!' said Sally. 'Who's a lucky boy, then?'

'I thought it only right to tell her about the Skidway Otter,' I said. 'It was the decent thing to do.'

As we left the ward the sister stopped us.

'We should have a pretty good record of how her brain is behaving,' she told me. 'It will be interesting to see if we can find anything out.'

It was a good job they had removed the wires before she opened her locker in the morning and found the burgundy nightdress – that would have recorded a seven on the Richter scale.

7

As I pulled the car to a halt outside my mother's house I knew that she was out shopping. It's funny, isn't it? Before you knock or ring the bell, you can tell that a house is empty. It has that feel about it.

It didn't really matter, she would be back soon. She always did her shopping in heats during the day, checking back every hour or so to see if the cat was all right. The final would be run around teatime. I could let myself in. She always left the key for me – in the lock where I could find it – and there was golf on television and there would be coffee in the jar marked flour. I pushed open the kitchen door and watched as the breadbin bounced jauntily across the lino tiles.

It was an old enamel breadbin, shaped like a roll-topped desk, with a front lid that folded inside itself. My mother had discovered that, no matter how she shook it, she could never clear out all the crumbs – no matter how she tried, the crumbs would hide in the corners, eventually turning a delightful fluorescent green.

When she bought a more conventional bin that could be flushed under the tap as God intended, she presented the old one to Whisky. He had always had an eye for gadgets and he commandeered the bread-bin as his sleeping quarters. My mother placed it between the fridge and the washing machine, and always left it with the lid rolled back. Whenever Whisky fancied forty winks, he simply nipped into his breadbin and jumped up and down a lot. Eventually, after a minute or two of violent leaping and cavorting, the lid would slam shut and the cat, by now completely knackered, settled down.

Cut off from the outside world and safe from any marauding mouse, he presumably dreamed that he was halfway across Europe, snuggled down in an upper berth on the Orient Express. His only problem was that, so far, he hadn't discovered any satisfactory way of getting himself *out* of the bread-bin. Since it must have been pitch-black in there and he was still saving for an alarm clock, he had no idea what time of day it was. So his only recourse was to attract attention to his plight by jumping up and down all over again and making a tremendous racket.

The Orient Express had been stopped by line repairs on the skirting board, and so I bent and rolled the lid back. Presumably Whisky had his eyes tight shut and, not registering that he had been released, was still frantically belting up and down. Eventually he realized that it had gone all light and he blinked and, giving me an embarrassed grin, staggered out to join the outside world.

★

I made a coffee, and Whisky and I settled down to watch the golf. These little breaks were a substitute for a lunch hour and Nick often joined me. With Sally at home I had been able to get in to the factory early, the result being that a brand-new design of French knicker, complete with cotton gusset, had just rolled off the production line. It was something to celebrate.

Whisky didn't care for golf and was soon bored – he preferred football and so I hurled his ping-pong ball around the room and he chased it. His control was good, his technique indifferent, and every foray ended with the ball, and Whisky's head, stuck underneath the settee. For the umpteenth time I was hauling him out by the back legs when my mother appeared. She plonked her shopping on the settee.

'Have you been here long?'

'No – ten minutes or so.'

'I wasn't in.'

'I thought that might be the case when you weren't here.'

'I was out.'

'That would account for it, then.'

You know – when people say that the art of conversation is dead, they just don't know what they are talking about.

The front doorbell dinged and my mother froze. She was always suspicious of the phone and of anyone who appeared at the front door. One evening I must have rung her a dozen times without getting an answer, and yet I knew she would be in. I began to imagine her lying on the bathroom floor in a coma, and around midnight I pulled the car out of the garage and set out on the twenty-five-mile round trip to see if she was all right.

When I burst in she was watching the late-night film on television.

'I've been ringing all night.'

'I know – that phone's never stopped.'

'Well, why didn't you answer it?'

'I would – but you never know who it's going to be, do you?'

I left, half relieved that she was safe and half wishing I'd found her in a coma on the bathroom floor.

She was just as wary of the front door, and now I watched as she moved sideways down the hall – one eye on the security chain and one ear cocked for sounds of movement. A man from Rotary had suggested the security chain and offered to fit it free, so she had taken him up on the offer.

She put one hand on the chain and an ear to the door.

'Who is it?'

It was Nick – I could see him as plain as day since the door was a sheet of clear glass. He was standing on the step looking in my mother's right ear.

'It's me.'

'Oh!'

The chain was flushed from its moorings and the door flung wide open.

'Oh, it's you!'

It's just a matter of knowing the password, you see. If the Black Panther or Jack the Ripper had said, 'It's me', they would have been welcome to come in and watch the golf or help pull the cat's head out from under the settee.

'If you're so careful about the front door, why do you leave the key in the back?'

She gave me one of her wily looks.

'Ah, but you see – there's only you who knows it's there.'

We watched the golf for a time and Nick and I chatted, except when the players were putting and the stewards held up placards asking for quiet. Then my mother made us shut up in case it put them off.

She couldn't get as enthusiastic about the golf as she did with the wrestling on a Saturday afternoon. Then, for an hour around teatime, Whisky was expected to wriggle out of her half nelsons and her flying buttocks as she tried to pin him to the rug.

However, she attempted to show some interest.

'Isn't that little Harry Carpenter?'

'Yes.'

'I thought he did the boxing.'

'He does the boxing as well,' Nick agreed.

'He'll get much more fresh air with the golf.'

She was pleased for Harry, and she offered other profound remarks as the players made their way up the fairway. Remarks such as: 'I don't know who buys his trousers but they've got no taste', and 'He picked the ball up then and I'm sure it wasn't his.'

It was a pleasant interlude, but it was time to be off. Then my mother said to Nick, 'I've just been to the chiropodist's to have my eyes tested.'

This was too good to miss, so we sat down again.

'That would make a nice change for him,' said Nick.

My mother settled down, glad to be rid of the golf and ready for a proper chat.

'He was very pleasant. He asked me what idiot had sold me my last pair of glasses.'

I could sense trouble. 'What did you tell him?'

'I told him *he* had.'

Now this wasn't really fair on the chiropodist. He had prescribed the glasses but they were for my father, and when he had died, some fourteen years ago, my mother had adopted them because she said they said they suited her better than her own. She'd bought hers from Woolworth's when she was sixteen.

'I asked him if I could have some contact lenses, but he thought I was too old to change now.'

I said, 'He's probably right.'

My mother wasn't so sure. 'Well, Minnie Bonsall wears them. Mind you – they've stuck hers right on her eyeballs. They shouldn't do that, should they?'

Nick shrugged. 'I suppose all you can do is put yourself in the hands of the chiropodist and trust him. You went with Minnie, did you?'

'Yes – and Nellie Elliot. Nellie's got a cataract.'

For a moment I had an awful feeling that she might have asked him if she could have a pair of cataracts as well – but no.

'He suggested a pair of bi-focals. They're very good – you can read a book and look at your feet at the same time.' And with that she opened her bag and took out a pair of spectacles.

'You haven't got them already?'

'Oh no! It'll take about a fortnight. These are Minnie's – she doesn't need them now she's got her contact lenses. In fact,' she said, getting up, 'I've half a mind to cancel mine – I can see perfectly well with these.'

She disappeared into the kitchen, and Nick and I tried not to look at one another. Nick picked up the passing Whisky and buried his face in his fur.

'Coffee?' My mother appeared at the doorway.

'Yes, thank you.'

'That would be very nice,' Nick approximated, spitting out hairs.

She turned and strode out to the kitchen, and then came the most awful crash as she went head over heels over the breadbin.

'You see,' she said as we picked her up, 'with the bi-focals I'd have seen that.'

We left her, unhurt and waving from the hallway.

Behind her in the kitchen we could see Whisky examining his breadbin and wondering whether or not to call in the builders.

Over the next week or so Diana slowly returned to her pre-fall condition. The EEG showed nothing and several other tests proved negative – they always did. On paper there was nothing wrong with her. Ed Boyle once wrote, 'Don't catch anything unless it is in the textbooks.' He was right, and the problem in neurology is that they are still writing the textbooks with stone chisels.

In the bed next to Diana was a delightful old lady who said to us, 'Do you realize that since we were admitted a week ago, sixteen people have been discharged – and not one of them was cured?'

Neurologists have problems. As consultants they feel the need to be as cocksure as consultants in other fields, and yet their science is so imprecise. However, they can't go home every night shouting, 'Hey – I've failed to diagnose thirty-nine people today.' They are getting well paid and their egos demand results, and so they fuel their diagnoses with a mixture of medical science and gut feeling. Very often they are wrong. I have sympathy for neurologists and yet, in most cases, a little humility might help. They can expect to retain the confidence of an intelligent and questioning patient for about eighteen months if they work at it. They often don the consultant's papal air of infallibility and appear to be the fount of all wisdom. This can work for many consultants in other fields – but the neurologist is rather like Tommy Docherty telling his footballers that they are the best in the world. After a while the patient begins to ask, 'Excuse me, boss – then why are we getting hammered week after week?'

A woman to whom none of this would be apparent simply appeared in the ward one day. Not from the world outside, but from the operating theatre. She was still under the effects of the anaesthetic as she was poured into the bed next to Diana and slept away the first few hours. That first night they forgot her pudding, but she didn't want to complain and it was left to Diana to point out to the nurses that she had missed the egg custard. Whether Diana did her a favour or not is open to question. Later her daughter and son-in-law visited and they talked quietly together, the three of them – not wanting to disturb anybody.

It was the following afternoon before Diana managed anything of a conversation with her new neighbour.

'Have you been in here before?'

'Yes.'

'What's the problem?'

'Multiple sclerosis.'

And that was that for the time being. The children came and went at visiting time, the Ovaltine was served, and it was under the cover of darkness that the woman offered: 'I found this lump.'

'In your breast?'

'Yes.'

'What did they say?'

'I came in for a test – a biopsy, they called it.'

'And what happened?'

'I don't know.'

She didn't know! She would have signed a form giving permission for the doctor to remove the breast if he thought it necessary, and she didn't know.

'Did you sign a form?'

'I think so.'

'Have you asked the nurses?'

'You don't like to, do you?'

She had obviously been brought to the neurological ward because she was an MS patient, otherwise she would have gone to a women's surgical unit. Something had gone wrong in the transfer and no one had told her – and you don't like to ask, do you?

'Would you like *me* to ask?'

'Oh, no – I'd rather you didn't. They've got enough on.'

Night passed and morning came and Diana probed further.

'Can you feel anything?'

'Not really.'

'Are you bandaged?'

'Yes.'

'Heavily bandaged, or is it just a strip?'

'There's quite a lot.'

'Look, let me tell the nurse.'

'No! Please. They'll tell me when they're ready.'

It was impossible to have even a quiet word with the nurse. The woman's pleading face begged her to be silent each time one approached.

Diana's chance came in the afternoon. The daughter brought two aunts with her, and whilst they were monopolizing her mother she turned to have a word with Diana.

'Look,' said Diana. 'Your mother has no idea whether she has had a mastectomy or not – will you tell the nurse?'

'Oh, I'm sure they'll tell her when they're ready.'

'She needs to know.'

'They know what they're doing – there's no need to bother them.' And with a patient smile she turned back to talk of other things.

Diana's sympathy was matched only by her fury at the family's submission. Eventually she was able to corner a nurse, who was appalled by the error. The woman's breast had been removed, together with much of the muscle on the chest wall.

My Auntie Jessie was once negotiating a zebra crossing when she was struck by a Chesterfield Corporation bus and lifted four feet through the air on to the far pavement.

She recovered consciousness as they were strapping her legs together, and the first thing she did was to apologize to the driver.

Diana was almost ready to come home. She was due to go down to the Maudsley soon, and any more tests would be conducted there. In the meantime she had been interviewed by a Dr Margaret something-or-other who had spent an hour or so with her, asking questions about her condition, her state of mind and how she coped.

'She was very pleasant. A bit wet behind the ears – but very pleasant.'

'What was she after?'

'Don't know. I think I'm a project – she wants to see you.'

Diana was perched on top of the bed covers, the now hip-length burgundy nightdress inching its way towards the bedhead.

I leaned forward in my chair and rested my chin on the bed.

'Do you realize that if a doctor did this he could see your pubic hairs?'

'He's already seen them.'

'One who hasn't.'

'Then I should do this.' She cracked me on the back of the neck with Fred's plastic hand and my adam's apple shot across into my left ear.

'When does this doctor want to see me?' I asked, wiping the tears from my eyes.

'You're to arrange it with the sister.'

The next afternoon Dr Margaret was waiting for me. She took me into a small office and sat me in a chair whilst she towered above me, legs swinging from a desk.

For the next hour she encouraged me to talk. Her questions were rather naïve – as though taken from course notes – and I tried to explain the less obvious problems of a relatively young woman who finds herself disabled.

She seemed more interested in me and my problems. How did I manage without sex? When told that I didn't manage without and, although it was different, it was extremely rewarding, she seemed surprised and wanted to know more.

I explained to her, in more detail than I shall do here, how it was possible to make sure that Diana bore no weight whatsoever and how, by monitoring her eyes, I was able to keep a check on her pain level. This meant a certain detachment on my part, but to give pleasure can often be more gratifying than to take it, and whatever our lovemaking lacked in spontaneity it more than made up for in ingenuity.

Making love to Diana took time. I once missed a whole cup final including extra time, the medal ceremony and the dressing room interviews. As a pain killer, sex was more effective than a hot bath – but since she often needed three hot baths a night, it was hardly likely to take over the number one spot as a palliative.

I explained how stress exhausted her. How the kids and I filtered all the bad news before it reached her – she was better at solving problems than the three of us put together, but it wore her out and since she could always trace a financial headache or my inability to meet a deadline back to her own condition, then it was better either to solve it first or, failing that, sweep it under the carpet.

I went on at length – too long. Dr Margaret was pleasant – too pleasant, as I told her of my life with Diana.

'She's a wonderful embroideress.'

'Oh.'

'No, not "Oh" – it's not a matter of the "Home Sweet Home" stuff. Diana's are modern embroideries – works of art. She sells them for a lot of money. She used to complete about one a month – now they take a year or more.'

'How does she manage with her hands?'

'She holds the needle between her second and third finger – then as she tires she uses pliers, held between her palms, and pulls the needle through with her teeth. If I'm there – I push it back.'

We talked – no, I talked, about my role in her life.

'Don't you sometimes resent having to do all this?'

'Yes – sometimes for as long as ten minutes. Then I watch her take a mug between her wrists and drink, or catch a glimpse of her face as she concentrates on her toes and wills them to move.'

She nodded – she seemed to understand.

A couple of days later the call came – we could take her home. Sally and I went through the house in a mist of Sparkle, Pledge and Windolene. Nick acted in an advisory capacity. He would lie on our bed, in the bath or on the sunbed, in any position that the horizontal Diana might take up on her return home, and he would imperiously point out to us the odd cobweb or mislaid slice of toast and marmalade.

During those periods when Diana was cocooned in her bedroom, we always tried to keep the house as clean and tidy as in the days when she was fit and well. It was impossible – without any apparent effort she could catch dust before it settled, and any spider who moved in with us was immediately trained to clean up after itself.

But we tried, and by and large we were reasonably successful. I changed from being a sloppy husband into a sloppy, houseproud husband, and Sally miraculously transmuted from slut to sloppy daughter. Nick acted in an advisory capacity.

It was important that we tried. It mattered to Diana that her house was neat and tidy, and the disabled are in an invidious position. She couldn't do it herself, and so she depended upon us. The alternative would have been for her either to plead or to nag, and so we happily scrubbed and scoured and made a point of reporting upstairs each stage of our sanitation programme, so that we could be patted on the head like puppies.

She could then receive visitors in her bedroom, knowing that on their way up through the house they would have smelt beeswax and fresh flowers.

Her opening remark would always be the same.

'I'm sorry the house is such a mess.'

Sally and I would glance at one another and then retire downstairs to discuss the various ways of strangling her.

I heaved the suitcase out of the car and dragged it screaming through the hospital reception area. A couple of other husbands, intent on evacuating their wives, carried empty suitcases lightly between forefinger and thumb.

My empty suitcase was packed with French knickers, waist slips, nightdresses and briefs. Diana always conducted a low-key selling campaign throughout her last days in a hospital, during which time the nurses took samples home to show friends and family.

Each nurse received a free pair of French knickers and a waist slip – the remainder were sold at cost price. My trade customers were crying out for supplies in the run-up to Christmas, but Diana insisted: 'We're talking pound notes here.'

I always lost money. Apart from the free gifts, the goods for nurses not on duty were left for them to collect and very rarely paid for. It would have been cheaper to join BUPA, but, as Diana said: 'Every little helps.'

I watched as she excitedly organized the distribution. She had notes of who wanted this and who wanted that, and money was being thrust in her direction. The underwear was laid out on her bed and the nurses and walking wounded crowded around her to claim their orders.

She couldn't cope. A year ago she would have taken it all in her stride – now she had difficulty adding up three items.

'Shall I deal with the money?'

She smiled at me. 'Right! Deric will take the money. Now – Christine! . . .'

Afterwards we sat in the patients' television room studying her orders. The consultant wanted to see her before she was discharged, and we spent the time balancing the books.

'You should have £57.30.'

I had £32.90. 'Yes – right on the button.'

'Worth the trouble, wasn't it?'

'You can say that again.'

The consultant studied Diana's medical notes and I studied the consultant. He was a good man – very highly thought of by his peers. He had been commended by the neurologists in London and, to his credit, had never minded us seeking answers elsewhere. He was somewhat aloof – even more distant in the hospital than he was at his home, but, although he kept one at arm's length, he was a gentle, kindly man whom Diana trusted.

The tests had proved nothing, as we had suspected, and he would be interested to see what the Maudsley had to say. He was closing the folder when Diana asked, 'What did the other doctor have to say?'

He sighed, as though expecting the question, and reopened the folder.

'It's rather long and complicated.'

'Her conclusions, then.'

The consultant flipped through three or four pages without reading them. Dr Margaret had been busy.

'She makes several points.'

'Such as?'

He leaned back in his chair. He didn't want to say this.

'Basically, she thinks that your problems are due to hysteria.'

We were silent. I can never remember us being so silent. Then Diana, staring down unbelievingly at her crumbling hands, said, 'She thinks it's all in my head?'

'She feels your problem has a psychoneurotic origin.'

For a moment Diana floundered, tears washing her eyes. For years the crippling disease now known as myalgic encephalomyelitis was dismissed as a purely hysterical illness – God knows what that diagnosis did to the poor souls who suffered from it.

'She's wrong,' I told him. 'I know Diana too well.'

'I think you're right,' he agreed. 'I know Diana rather well myself.'

'Then why . . .?'

'The doctor is young. She still thinks there's an answer to everything – it would be important to her to . . . er . . . to impress me.'

'She doesn't impress me,' muttered Diana. 'I want those notes removed from my file.'

'I'm sorry – I can't do that.'

Diana was beginning to fight back. 'If that stays in my file it will colour everyone's opinion from here on. Every ward sister will read that I'm just a hysterical woman, and that's just how they will treat me.'

'Oh, I don't think so.'

'I do – it's an easy answer and they'll latch on to it.'

He stared at the file and jabbed the offending pages with his biro.

'Much as I disagree with her opinion, it would be professionally unethical for me to remove a colleague's notes from your file.'

'It wouldn't if I did it,' said Diana.

'Other doctors won't know that she's young and inexperienced,' I pointed out. 'They might take it as a mature opinion.'

Diana eased her wheelchair back. 'I want it out.'

The consultant considered first me and then the file. He leaned forward, chin on hands, and spoke to Diana. 'I understand, but I just can't help you. Perhaps you could do *me* a favour,' and handing the file to Diana he asked, 'Would you be so kind as to hand this in at reception on your way out?'

As the wheelchair bounced along the corridor Diana clutched the case notes fiercely to her breast. I was silent. It's not easy at the best of times to hold a conversation with the back of a head – right now the words wouldn't come.

Diana signalled for me to slow down. 'I'll go in there,' she said, pointing to the toilet for the disabled.

That is often easier said than done. Sometimes, when it has been adapted from an ordinary toilet, the space between the two sets of doors doesn't allow for a wheelchair and a minder, and if you have ever sat in a wheelchair and tried to open a door marked 'Pull' then you have attempted the impossible.

We managed, and I hung around outside trying not to look furtive. Time passed, and twice I nipped back in to see if all was well. My enquiries were both met with a grunt that said, 'Yes – push off. I'll tell you when.'

Eventually there was a banging of wheelchair against wood and I opened the doors and hauled her out. She was hunched in the chair, a sure sign that the pain was taking control once more, and we moved towards the exit. The sooner we were home the better.

The nurse on duty at the desk was half hidden behind a mound of files, her face harassed and her hair escaping from beneath a crisp but cock-eyed hat.

I slowed to a halt and reached for the file on Diana's lap. I looked at the face in the wheelchair and raised my eyebrows – Diana nodded and I dropped the bundle on to the desk with a thump.

I swung the car into the traffic and headed for home. We didn't talk. Our heads were full with random bits and pieces all tumbling over one another and with half-thoughts and strips of conversation fighting for pride of place at the front. As we left the city behind us and touched the moors leading into Baslow, Diana opened the *Woman's Own* that she had stolen from the ward. She took out four sheets of paper and began to read.

She read slowly, going back now and then to the previous page. I waited. There's a time to talk and a time to shut up – this was a time to shut up. She had been hurt more than when they had to break her fingers, and any platitudes that I had at the ready were better left unwrapped.

'The bitch – the little bitch.'

'She was a very young bitch.'

'She should have been strangled at birth.'

'Wet behind the ears – remember?'

She read on until I pulled into the drive. I switched off the engine and waited. Perhaps Diana knew we had arrived home – perhaps she didn't. The back door opened and Sally and Nick appeared, grinning. I nodded a warning to them and the grins dropped off and the door closed.

'How did you tear them out?'

'I opened the file, knelt on it and pulled the pages out between my wrists – one at a time.'

'Can we get rid of them?'

She stared down at the sheets of paper.

'You don't think that, do you – that it's all in my head?'

'Never. Not for a single moment have I ever thought that.'

'And this won't make any difference?'

'You know it won't. I love you.''

I took the pages from her knee and screwed them up in a ball.

'Come on – let's go in.'

She smiled. The hurt wasn't over – it would go on for a long time, coming back at odd moments to nag away at her. To be doubted, to be told by those you thought to be on your side that the wasted legs, the skeletal hands and the pain that had taken over your life were a product of something inside your own head was cruel, and brought with it its own pain.

107

But she smiled and said, 'She thinks that you are an over-anxious husband.'

'She doesn't?'

'She does.'

'The little bitch.'

My mind flipped back to the early hours of a cold morning. Diana was soaking in her third bath of the night and I was tired and curled up on the bathroom floor. My eyes were heavy and for a few moments I dropped off to sleep. Something woke me and I couldn't see Diana – I scrambled to the edge of the bath to find her lying, not breathing, on the bottom.

I raised her into a sitting position and held her tight. Her eyes were shut and her head did an untidy balancing act on her neck. I did nothing – I couldn't think, I just held her and slowly the eyes opened and took in their surroundings. She hadn't taken a single breath – God knows how long she had been under water.

'I went, didn't I?'

'You blacked out – just for a moment.' And in that moment I could have lost her.

'How silly – why is my hair wet?'

An over-anxious husband? Now why, I wonder, could Dr Margaret possibly think that?

8

It was just like the old days, except that the Fine Fare supermarket hadn't been there in the old days. I pushed the trolley and Sally dropped things into it. Then I looked at the prices and put them back on the shelves.

'Do you still eat tinned baby foods?' I asked her.

'Don't be so daft.'

'It's no good looking at me like that. You were still buying a tin of apple dessert every week when you were twenty-one.'

'I haven't had one for ages,' she said, plucking a tin of beef and bone hotpot from the shelf and tossing it into the trolley.

'What's this, then?' I asked, picking up the little red tin with its picture of a bouncing baby.

'That is *junior* beef and bone hotpot – the baby food is in blue tins.' And with that she added a tin of junior cherry and banana yoghurt and wandered over to the frozen chickens.

For a moment I considered buying her a packet of Pampers. They were on special offer and I wondered if we would need fresh supplies of Milton to sterilize her bottle for the few more days she would be with us.

To her credit, my twenty-four-year-old daughter didn't stamp her foot at the checkout when she saw the chocolate buttons, and so I bought her a packet of Jellitots and she sucked them contentedly all the way home.

Nick's new car was parked outside the house, and Sally raced in to give him a hug as I hauled in the carrier bags. We go in for a lot of hugging in our house – it never did anyone any harm.

I could hear them chatting away in the lounge. Sally about her interview with the Tao Clinic in Leicester, and Nick about the house he was proposing to buy in Darley Dale.

They were both doing well, and my mind flipped back to the days when they would rush home, still muzzy from the classroom, and chat away to Diana for what seemed like hours, until they had worked school right out of their system. It was good to see them now, grown up and independent.

Suddenly I heard Nick ask, 'What time is it?'

'It's a quarter to two,' Sally told him and I thought, 'He must have an appointment. Probably quite an important one by the sound of it – some deal he's cooking up.'

'Quick!' I heard him cry. 'It's " Postman Pat".' Sally shot across to the television, and within seconds the tune 'Postman Pat, Postman Pat, Postman Pat and his black and white cat' came rippling into the kitchen. I put my head round the door and peeped at them before I went upstairs to see Diana.

'Aren't they grown up?' She pointed to the shiny white car standing proudly at the top of the drive. 'They haven't had it easy, but they've both worked really hard – it seems only yesterday that they were just a couple of little kids who could hardly carry their satchels. What are they doing now?'

'They are both sitting on a cushion on the floor,' I told her. 'He's eating a tin of junior cherry and banana yoghurt – she's eating a tin of junior beef and bone hotpot, and they're watching Postman Pat and his black and white cat on the television.'

'It's not that time already, is it?' cried Diana, jabbing at her remote control thingy.

'Damn – I've missed the beginning,' she grumbled, and I crept out of the room as Postman Pat put on his roller skates and went to find the vicar to tell him that his sister was coming up to see him and he didn't have to go down to London after all.

There were times when I wondered if I was the only grown-up in the house, and especially so that night, as I crept into Sally's room to kiss her good night. She was tucked up cosy and warm, and sharing her bed, his head on the pillow, was Adrian the three-foot-tall teddy bear who was just a few months younger than Sally herself.

She woke as I kissed her. 'You big softie,' she murmured, half asleep. 'It's a long time since you kissed me good night.'

I didn't tell her that I always popped into her bedroom last thing at night, even when she wasn't there.

Nothing to do with sentiment, you understand – nothing like that. It's just that I thought it only right and proper to see that Adrian, who spent his days chatting to Duncan the yellow elephant on the wooden chest, should spend his nights tucked up warm and cosy, nearest side to the wall, in Sally's bed.

You know – just for old times' sake.

Diana had just moved into a spell of blessed remission. Every now and then, perhaps once a year, a strange wave of dizzyness would sweep over her. It was like nothing else – her head would wheel and whirl and become so light that she could feel each hair floating.

'It's as though the most wonderful anaesthetic has been injected into the base of my skull.'

Then, within the hour, all the strings of her body, the tendons and sinews would relax and stretch and the pain would withdraw, standing off at a bearable level.

It would be back with a vengeance. These remissions were getting shorter, and the hands would remain clawed and the legs more or less useless – but for a while she could sample a life where stirring a cup of tea wasn't a major exercise of will.

We have all seen the wheelchair athletes, those who throw the javelin, hurl the discus and catapult their wheelchairs towards the finishing tape. It takes a tremendous amount of iron will and courage, but very often the only difference between them and the hunched up creature in the corner being talked at in a loud voice is the pain. Constant pain brings with it an overwhelming exhaustion, and the exhaustion, in turn, brings yet more pain. This was something we had to watch with Diana. Take the remission for granted, and it was over.

Elkie Brooks was singing 'Lilac Wine' when it happened, and I was accompanying her on the spoons. To Elkie's credit she didn't let it put her off, but Diana was already winding up Fred's trusty right hand. She caught me a powerful blow on the back of the knees, and whenever she did that it was a sure sign of disapproval. As I searched for my lead spoon under the wardrobe I heard a deep sigh from the bed and, as I watched, the injection began to work and the hair began to float and the sinews relaxed and unwound.

The next afternoon found us retracing the steps Sally and I had taken through the new Fine Fare supermarket in Matlock. Not perhaps one of the most exciting jaunts on which we could have embarked, but Diana had never been inside the store and it was close to home in case this pain-free interlude proved to be a false alarm.

One of the great advantages of a supermarket is that the aisles are wide enough to accommodate a wheelchair. Many cute little shops are a no-go area with their split-level floors and their fancy displays.

We had already made a dummy run into Woolworth's which came to nothing, thanks to that rare and wonderful British institution – the helpful shop assistant. As we approached the glass doors, the young man was fastening a 'That's the wonder of Woolies' sticker to the glass. In a matter of seconds he was pulling up a brass bolt and had the double doors thrown open wide enough to accommodate a Sherman tank. We thanked him graciously as we passed through and made for the Do-It-Yourself section at the far end of the store. Suddenly I panicked – I always do when I realize that I haven't a single cigarette about my person – and I swung the chair around and made for the kiosk near the entrance.

The young man saw us coming and, leaping from his steps, he yanked out the bolt and flung the doors wide open, shouting, 'Just a moment, please' to several would-be customers who were about to enter. It would have been churlish to let him down, and so I adjusted the course of the chair by a few degrees and we sailed through the doors and out on to the cold pavement. As we passed, I thanked the assistant wholeheartedly, whilst Diana gave a Queenly wave and a nod to those lined up on either side of the doors.

There were no such problems in the supermarket – the doors were automatic and programmed to obey. We were in no hurry, and stopped every few yards to chat to friends we hadn't seen in a while. The conversations were hardly earth-shattering, but we enjoyed them.

'How old will your Eric be now, then?'

'She's run off with who?'

'Of course I could see it coming a mile off.'

'A grandmother! You never are? You haven't changed a bit.'

You know the sort of thing – and very pleasant it was, too. We must have been in the shop for almost an hour and the wire basket was still empty, so we decided to start flinging a few goodies into it before the management threw us out.

I took my place in the queue at the bacon counter, and Diana decided to set off on a journey into the unknown and investigate the yoghurts. I had told her about the yoghurt – they sold it in huge gallon buckets and it had amused me to see, written on the lid, 'Eat within two days.' I reckoned that if you ate your way through a gallon of yoghurt in two days you would never want to look another yak in the face as long as you lived. So Diana set off to see if I had been exaggerating. I had, of course, but they *were* big buckets, and she disappeared around a burial mound of Persil Automatic to investigate.

It took ages before I was served at the bacon counter. I didn't know that they had one of those ticket machines out of which you must first pluck a number. I must have said 'Excuse me. I was here first' a dozen times before a small child in a push-chair put me right.

Clutching my bacon and a small plastic beaker full of cockles I set off in the general direction of the yoghurt. She had obviously tired of that particular section. I suppose there is a limit to the time you can spend being enthralled by a display of yoghurt – even if it is packed in big buckets – and I moved on to wine and spirits.

If you lose a partner in our supermarket it isn't too difficult to locate them. All you have to do is stand still and pivot through a range of 360 degrees until you see the head you are looking for over the top of the fixtures. But it isn't that easy when your partner is in a wheelchair – they are too low down. The only way you are ever going to find them is to belt up and down each and every aisle and hope that eventually you will come across them. I had no luck at all, and I was standing back at the bacon counter, hoping that Diana might come looking for me, when a very sweet old lady came bowling up from the bakery end.

'Is anything wrong?' she asked kindly. I must have looked perturbed – the over-anxious husband.

'I've lost my wife,' I told her, and she touched my arm.

'I lost my husband in 1968,' she murmured. 'Never had a day's illness in his life.' And she went on to tell how things would never be the same again, but I must soldier on.

116

The more she sympathized, the more impossible it became for me to explain that Diana and I had merely become separated in the store. I listened for several minutes more and then, out of the corner of my eye, spotted the wheelchair nosing its way around the fresh cream cakes. I raised my eyebrows and signalled with my eyes for Diana to pass on by. With an understanding born of over twenty-five years of marriage she paddled on towards the mixed pickles as though she had never seen me before in her life.

We met up again in pet foods and cereals. She was piled high with giant cornflake packets, kitchen rolls, toilet rolls, bread rolls and a huge bucket of yoghurt. A Pickford's truck would have been more appropriate than a wheelchair.

She had a love-hate relationship with the wheelchair. Without it, of course, life would have been impossible, but she could never get used to staring at navels all day. One remedy was to turn the chair into a chariot. As we left the checkout, Diana would shout 'Charge!' and I would take a good long run and, gathering up a head of steam and a little bit of speed, we would charge at the automatic doors.

The last few strides are electric. The hair stands on end, and a tingle from head to foot tells you that this time they are not going to open. But so far they always had, and we hurtled through out on to the pavement. One day, perhaps, we would try and go through a door marked 'Entrance only' and finish

117

up a tangled mess of glass, limbs and yoghurt. I didn't quite know how I would explain it all to the management.

'The brakes failed as we went past the Shreddies.'

'We hit a patch of black ice just by the Branston pickle.'

The true answer, I suppose, would have to be, as with caves and mountains, 'Because it was there.'

That Saturday Sally was due to leave for Leicester. She had arranged a bed sitting room for herself – "£12 a week with garden view." I was more than a little suspicious about this room.

'It's adequate,' Sally offered. 'Leicester is very reasonable.'

For twelve pounds a week she was more likely to be in the garden itself, and she certainly wasn't too anxious for me to see it.

'It has a bed and a chest of drawers and . . . I think there's a chair, I'm not sure.'

I was determined to see this room.

Diana was not coming with us. She had wanted to, but a week of small adventures had left her exhausted and she needed to rest. I was relieved. If the room was as bad as we expected, I would be able to lie about it.

As Sally packed, I soaked in the bath and examined my thighs. Once they had been footballer's thighs, thick and solid. Now I could wrap both hands around them. I weighed myself, and the needle settled just below the eight stone mark. For twenty years I had weighed a steady ten and a half, but over the past twelve months the weight had dropped off. Two and a half stone in under a year. The doctor had said it was worry – at this rate I should disappear before I was fifty.

There was a knock at the door and Sally burst in, shouting, 'Are you decent?'

I wasn't, but I did the best I could with a small brown flannel the size of a postage stamp.

'Good God!' she cried. 'You look like a cross between Mahatma Gandhi and an oven-ready chicken.'

She scooped up an armful of smelly things and departed, leaving me to examine the evidence in the steamy mirror.

Tony Curtis did not look back at me as he had when I was a youth, and Charles Bronson, who had appeared in the mirror as the lines began to etch deep in my face, was no longer there. I thought I caught a glimpse of Old Man Steptoe leering through the steam, and I quickly dressed and tried to think of other things.

Sally was on the phone to my mother as I carried her case downstairs. Teddy bear Adrian and Duncan the yellow elephant were waiting for me in the hall, wearing silly smiles and guarding half our kitchen utensils packed in cardboard boxes.

My mother was wishing Sally well.

'Where will you be living?'

'Not far from the cricket ground.'

'Oh, you'll like that.'

My mother always made a point of half-researching anything that interested the children. Sally was a cricket fanatic.

'Doesn't David Gower play for Leicester?'

'That's right – I'm in love with David Gower.'

'He hasn't done too well lately, has he?'

'Oh I don't know – a hundred and two yesterday.'

'Oh, well. There's no wonder. Not with a temperature like that.'

There *was* a chair in the room, a stick insect of a chair, and it looked marginally more comfortable than the bed. As we had entered the large Victorian house the smell of damp and decay had assaulted my senses, and my heart fell as we trooped along an artificial corridor, erected from hardboard and designed to mask any elegance the house might have once possessed. Down four steps and along another corridor was Sally's room – tucked away in the basement of the house, as though it were ashamed of itself. I dropped the case to the floor and looked about me. It was little wider than the corridor, and just a little longer than it was wide. Sally began to bustle.

'When I get my posters up . . . .'

At the far end of the room, although the room was too small to have a far end, was a glass door.

French window would be too grand a term. The garden was overgrown and threatening to invade the room, and either the house had sunk or the garden had been raised, because a foot of soil was stacked against the bottom two panes of the door.

Kneeling down, I could see a cross-section of soil through the glass, and I watched fascinated as a worm looked in to get a glimpse of the new tenant.

'Well – what do you think?'

I thought it was very close to my idea of hell, except that hell was hardly likely to be damp.

'It's a bit damp.'

'Oh well, my fan heater will soon fix that.' Sally was in that sparky sort of mood which promotes instant action, anything to drive away the thought that all this might be a mistake.

'At least I have two doors in case of fire.'

You couldn't have set that room alight with a blowtorch. The wallpaper stood away from the wall as though allergic to plaster, and when we pointed the fan heater at the bed, the glass door steamed up.

'Let me show you the kitchen.'

The kitchen was unremarkable, but not so the three girls sitting around the table drinking coffee. They were bright and friendly and generated a wartime spirit against a common enemy – the landlord.

'If we were gerbils the RSPCA would have him put away for life.'

As the horror stories unfolded we became caught

up in an effervescent mood of rebellion. Living in a damp cell could be fun as long as you had someone to hate. We listened as they plotted to kill the girl on the first floor – the one who had the best room, the room in which you could sleep without an overcoat. Sally's spirits soared, and by the time we introduced Adrian the teddy bear and Duncan the yellow elephant to the bedsit we were almost able to persuade them that they were taking a step up in the world.

9

The next couple of weeks were exceptional in that they were almost normal, and Diana beamed through the whole fortnight. Every now and then, when her back was turned, Dr Margaret's words would steal in amongst her thoughts and catch her unawares, but a steady stream of visitors flowed up the stairs bearing gifts and gossip to drive them away again.

Between them her friends organized 'Diana Watch', so that I could nip down to London for two days. Rosie would help with her embroidery and talk and chat. Rosie was no mean embroideress herself, and an acknowledged expert at talking and chatting. Myrna would bring flowers from her shop and stay, pretending that she wasn't busy. Margaret, our friendly local chemist and recent neighbour, would spread perfumes all over the bed pretending they were free samples. Gill would bring chocolates from Harrods and scatter them as though they were Smarties. She was better known by Harrods than I was by Mr Windley of the Matlock Green Army Stores. Nick would take over the night shift, and I would worry because I knew I was indispensable.

★

I had six talks to record for 'Woman's Hour' and a piece for 'Does He Take Sugar?' I also wanted to snatch the opportunity to see old friends and meet Kay Evans of 'Woman's Hour' for the first time. Kay and I had corresponded for years, ever since her first rejection had landed on my mat. I had recorded a Christmas piece for the programme and she was not impressed.

' . . . *Although I liked your style of writing and presentation, I am afraid that the overall effect was patronizing; I doubt if our audience would enjoy the basic premise that your wife would have shown so little interest in the Christmas dinner that she would have left the choice of bird in the hands of an evident incompetent. Christmas is a hard market to break into, you know, and only very good material stands a chance.*'

'Up yours,' I thought as I tossed the letter into the wastepaper basket. Then, having played the tape over, I fished the letter out of the basket and ironed it carefully with my hand. Kay wasn't to know that this evident incompetent had to do the Christmas shopping because his wife was ill – and if she didn't, neither would the listeners.

Since then she had accepted all my pieces, suggesting a little editing at first and then giving me my head as I adapted to the house style of the programme. We seemed to write every other week, and in our letters we discussed such topics as the inventor of the baked potato and the works of Petroleum V. Naseby, and insulted one another with a growing affection. I was looking forward to meeting her.

She was out. I chatted with a secretary who pretended to know who I was, and then I roamed all over Broadcasting House and got lost. I passed Norman Tebbit three times. He was being escorted by a white-faced young man who was obviously just as lost as I was, and then I went looking for the office of the Assistant to the Deputy Director General.

Roger Protheroe was filling this post for a spell and, since I was never likely to know another assistant to the Deputy Director General of the BBC, I was determined to seek him out.

He was in America. I passed Norman again on my way to Radio Two continuity where Paul Leighton spent his waking hours.

'He's in Matlock – he'll be back on Wednesday.'

'I shall be in Matlock then.'

Marlene Pease, the producer of 'Does He Take Sugar?', gave me coffee and a warm welcome. I suggested that maybe the title of her programme was just a mite sexist and could be changed, for six months of the year, to 'How Are Her Periods?' She said she would think about it, but she hasn't.

I nodded to my friend Norm as I left her office and went in search of Mike Ingham of 'Sport on Two'.

'He's in Belgrade – or somewhere. Shall I enquire?'

'No – Belgrade is far enough, thank you.'

It seemed that Broadcasting House was emptying

fast, and so I made my way over to Radio London to see Charles Murray.

'He's in the pub.' Knowing Charles, I should have gone there first. I tried three pubs, and three gin and tonics later I was back in my hotel talking to Diana on the phone.

'Are you having a good time?'

'Terrific.'

'What have you been doing?'

'I went for a walk with Norman Tebbit.'

She seemed to accept this as something that happened to you when you were in London. 'What are you doing tomorrow?'

'Going to see Neil Everton at Breakfast Television.'

'Give him my love.'

'I will.'

He was on holiday.

Diana was on a high and we made the most of it. Brian and Gill Money took us to a night club in Doncaster to see the Grapevine fashion show. Grapevine was a weird and wonderful shop, with an unusual approach to business, spelt out in the legend on its carrier bags – 'Paris, Milan and Tickhill'.

Brian bundled us out of the car outside the club and roared off to find a parking space – then the bouncers pounced. They reversed their usual procedure and tried to bounce Diana in.

'Leave it to us,' they cried with a confidence built

of raw muscle and, leaving me with the door swinging in my face, they kick-started her into the building.

Nothing is more terrifying to the occupant of a wheelchair than the sudden appearance of well-meaning amateurs. She hadn't encountered well-meaning gorillas before. Gill and I tumbled in through the door to see her being propelled across the foyer towards the foot of an enormous staircase. The bouncers paused, one either side the chair.

'No,' I shouted, but they didn't understand long words. They each took an arm of the chair and, in one graceful movement, lifted and launched themselves onwards and upwards.

They stopped somewhere around the third step. By this time they had realized that they looked somewhat silly, standing there, each holding just the side of a wheelchair.

Diana sat in the skeleton and waited for them to shuffle back down.

'Thank you, but I think I'll go up on my bum – could you give me a hand?' The chief bouncer handed his half of the chair to his assistant and, lifting her out, placed her gently on the stairs.

'Don't worry about the chair, it's always happening.'

Gill acted as her marshal and I set about putting the chair together again. The staircase seemed to go on for ever, and I watched as they slowly climbed towards a snow-capped chandelier.

She hated these public performances. She never felt less feminine than at times like this: feet on one step, miss a step, bottom on the next, then the elbow dug in the carpet to give purchase, a rolling heave and repeat it all over again. All around her people swarmed up the stairs. They were very good, they gave her plenty of room – too much room, as a thoughtful motorist might give a horse rider on a country lane. This left a dance floor for her to perform upon under the spotlight gaze of the crowd. She would have been hidden amongst a forest of legs, but, in her little clearing, she was on show and the often muttered, 'Poor thing!' did nothing to ease her discomfort.

We had tried every which way to conquer a long flight of stairs. Dragging the chair up backwards frightened the life out of both of us, and for me to carry her was just as hair-raising – one stumble in either case and the result didn't bear thinking about.

No, bum-travel was slow but sure. We had tried it once at the Buxton Opera House, and she had been so exhausted by the time she reached the summit that, after a rest on a couch, she had bummed it straight back down again and spent the following week in bed.

Brian joined us three-quarters of the way up the north face.

'Come on, Diana – stop arsing about.' He has a way with words.

Laughter cracked the reverential silence about us, and passers-by joined in with offers of help.

'I've got a tow rope in the car, love.'

Diana smiled, thankful to be out of the limelight and back in the chorus again.

During the next few days there were signs that the truce was almost over, and whatever this damned illness was it began sending out scouts to plan its next campaign.

Several times we attempted to go out – just for a spin around town in the chair – but the sheer effort of being dressed would exhaust her and, after a short spin around the bedroom instead, she would be back between the sheets – too tired to be disappointed.

The disappointment would harden as a trickle of energy returned, and it was then that she would brood over what was no longer possible in her life. At other times she would either be glorying in her new-found freedom or occupied completely in dealing with the pain and frustration.

But in this half-light she would get ratty and find fault with everything. I, on the other hand, would remain calm and serene, understanding that I had to be strong at this time and take the brickbats like a man.

'What's this?'

'Steak and kidney.'

'You could have fooled me.'

'You liked it last time.'

'I must have been delirious – what's that?'

'The rose off the watering can.'

'Why is it there?'

'I thought you'd like a rose on your tray.'

'Is that supposed to be a joke?'

'Yes.'

'Well, it's a stupid joke.'

'Just trying to cheer you up.'

'Well, don't.'

'All right, stuff it then – pardon me for breathing.'

Sometimes I could remain calm and understanding for at least two and half minutes, but that was on a good day.

The cold war period that usually follows an argument is especially cruel for the disabled. That heavy swirling silence, where thoughts tumble over one another behind a glowering mask – 'I'm not speaking until he does' – can only be maintained until they have to ask: 'Will you take me to the toilet, please?'

And then a body, stiff with indignation, must allow itself to be lifted and lowered and then framed by a lavatory seat. I only let it happen once, and I was ashamed of myself.

Saturdays were important to me. On behalf of BBC Radio Derby I travelled not quite the length, but definitely the breadth of England reporting on football matches. I enjoyed it – it brought a breath of fresh air, chilblains and the prospect of pneumonia into my life.

In the morning I cooked and cleaned and flew around the Matlock shops ticking off items from Diana's list. I was becoming a superb shopper and a first-rate wire basket handler. I could now ask for 'Ten Tampax Super, please' without stammering, and discuss intelligently the merits of Comfort fabric conditioner with any like-minded housewife. By eleven in the morning I would have a cold lunch for Diana hermetically sealed in clingfilm and placed on her bedside table along with fresh fruit and orange juice. Then we would have a coffee together before I plastered my limbs in thermal underwear and set forth in search of a far-off press box, set in a distant football ground.

That little dot which jumps up and down in an excited frenzy whilst printing out the football results on television would be flexing its muscles in readiness, determined to spell Hartlepool correctly this week, as I pulled into the fair city of Liverpool. Already the Everton coaches, blue and white scarves streaming from the windows, would be nosing into Newcastle, and here at home some forty thousand Liverpool fans marched on Anfield – a red and white army charged with enthusiasm and best bitter.

I sniffed the air, thick with anticipation, and then turned the car sadly in the direction of Holly Park, the home of South Liverpool Football Club – a sort of Stalag 7 with meat pies. Outside, a whole police-man was on duty as the Matlock Town fans, already half crazed on tepid Bovril, poured out from a ten-year-old Vauxhall Victor.

This was my Saturday afternoon. Two hours there, two hours back, and two hours spent fighting for a phone so that my live dispatches, via Radio Derby, would bring joy to the multitudes as they cleaned their cars or painted the back bedroom. I loved every minute of it. The sensual pleasures of Worksop one week – the erotic atmosphere of Goole the next. At Gainsborough a press box set high in the stand. Here at Holly Park, a phone strung halfway up the wall of a concrete bunker outside the dressing rooms – the cord not quite long enough to enable the commentator actually to see the match as he talked.

The enemy on these occasions were the local newspaper reporters, who treated the phone as though they had built it themselves out of milk bottle tops. Often as many as six of us fought over one phone. At first I had been polite and hesitant – now I was as ignorant as the rest of them. Here at South Liverpool the local newspaperman and I had an arrangement. I could use the phone whenever I wanted – otherwise I broke his neck. Unfortunately it wasn't possible to engage the telephone operator in hand to-hand-combat. After a five-minute wait, 'I want to reverse the charges on a call to Derby, and I don't want any pips please.'

'You've got to have pips.'

'No, I haven't.'

'You have.'

'I haven't – it's a commentary going out live on the radio. I don't want any pips.'

'You've got to have pips.'

'Can I speak to the supervisor, please.'

Another long wait. I stare at the concrete wall and the local reporter lowers his head ready to charge.

'Hullo?'

'I want to make a reverse call charge to Derby, and I don't want any pips.'

'You've got to have pips.'

'No, I haven't. I do this every week – time me on the clock.'

Eventually we reach agreement and I hear, 'I have a call for you from Liverpool. Will you accept the . . .'

'Yes,' butts in a studio voice. 'Where the hell have you been?'

As the programme comes live down the phone I hear a cheer from the other side of the bunker.

'What's happening?' I ask the reporter, but suddenly he's gone deaf. I haven't seen any football for ten minutes, and then a voice down the phone tells me: 'You're next.'

Steve Orme is on the line from Burton, and he winds up his report with: 'The corner came across, but he kept his head and volleyed it low into the far corner of the net . . .'

133

Alex Trelinski controls himself with difficulty as he announces, 'And now over to Deric Longden at South Liverpool.'

I can't control myself, even with difficulty, and precious seconds tick by as I fight with hysteria. 'Well no heads here being volleyed into the net, Alex – but Matlock came close to scoring in the third minute when . . . pip-pip-pip-pip.'

I developed a hatred of phones in those Northern Premier League days that I find hard to conquer even now. Once, at Southport, the telephones had been cut off because the club hadn't paid their bill, and as each deadline approached I had to sprint up the road and forcibly evict an old lady from a phone box as she spent the afternoon trying to ring her son in Grimsby. Four times this happened, and each time the gate man made me pay to get back into the ground.

On my way to Grantham one November Saturday, it became increasingly obvious that I would never reach the ground for the kick-off. A quarter of an hour after the start I was still miles away, and so I pulled into a Volvo garage and asked if I could use the phone.

'For the BBC – I'll reverse the charges.'

'By my guest.'

I waited silently for my introduction and then hurled myself into: 'It's been really end-to-end stuff so far this afternoon with neither team getting the upper hand. Matlock forced a corner in the first minute, but Grantham were soon on the attack and Wilson had to be quick off his line to tidy up what could have been a dangerous situation.' I carried on in this vein for a minute or so, ending with: 'The score here at Grantham: Grantham nil – Matlock nil. Now back to the studio.'

I thanked the salesman for the use of the phone.

'No trouble.'

'You got me out of a hole.'

'Don't mention it – but I'll never trust you buggers again.'

At the ground, with twenty-five minutes gone, I collared the man on the turnstile.

'What's the score?'

'Nil – nil.'

'Anything happened?'

'It's been end-to-end stuff, really. Matlock had a corner early on, but we should have scored straight after – your goalie had to be quick off his line.'

On Saturdays I could shut out all my worries and fears for an afternoon – drown them in Bovril, steep them in clichés and swathe them in thermal underwear, so that I could return home refreshed and ready to convince myself, all over again, that cooking, cleaning and nursing were all that I wanted to do with my life.

Diana was sitting up in bed, sandbagged in by

135

pillows as though she were manning a machine gun nest. Margaret was sitting in the line of fire, looking worried. I glanced at Diana's eyes as I kissed her cheek.

'Hullo, love – how have you been?'

'Fine.'

'She hasn't,' said Margaret. 'Something strange has been happening.'

Diana's eyes were a giveaway. Her eyeballs were black and dancing to a tune of their own.

'I'm all right. It's just my hands.'

'I've never seen anything like it,' said Margaret. 'I couldn't do anything – she's been so ill.'

'Don't worry, Margaret – it happens,' Diana told her, and the glance she gave me told me how pleased she was to have me home to share the pain. A one-second glance and it made everything worthwhile. 'It happens – doesn't it?'

'Yes,' I said, stroking her hair. 'Let's have a look at your hands.'

I raised the sheets gently and, taking her forearm, lifted her right hand on to a pillow.

The hand was clenched into a fist so tight that her arm was death-white from the elbow down and, having locked the fingers back on themselves, the arm had gone on twisting until her knuckles were hard against her wrist.

'It's impossible,' Margaret sobbed, tears running down her cheeks. She was trying to touch her own wrist with her knuckles. 'It's impossible.'

'It just happens,' Diana stared down at her arm, a touch of pride mixing in with the pain.

It had been a rough couple of hours for Margaret. As a chemist she was cool, calm and professional – as a woman she was highly emotional, and the chemist had called it a day. The woman was taking over and crying like a baby.

Diana had cried the first time, and not just from the pain. To watch your arm roll up like a hosepipe was unnerving, to say the least. I had panicked and, picking her up, rushed her down to the doctor's. He had sat and watched in amazement as the arm continued to fold. At the hospital the Casualty team sat and watched in amazement. I looked after her myself nowadays – I was perfectly capable of looking on in amazement.

The pattern was always the same. Whatever the force was that was torturing her in this way, it would now take a rest for a while and then return to work on her upper arm.

I was wet through with sweat. The thermal underwear that had defeated the concrete chill and icy winds of Liverpool was becoming squishy in the heat of the bedroom.

'Can you hang on for a moment, Margaret? While I get my coat off.'

I popped into Sally's room and peeled off the outer layers until the snow-white vest and pale pink longjohns were exposed.

Sally had once washed a thermal vest for me and

137

then committed it to the tumble dryer – now Adrian the teddy bear wore it on cold nights in Leicester, and it was rather tight on him.

When she had washed the longjohns she told me, 'Do you want the good news or the bad news?'

'The good.'

'They haven't shrunk.'

'And the bad?'

'They've gone pink.' I would have died had anyone seen me in them.

I didn't die when Margaret walked into the bedroom. I simply turned the same colour as the pants. But Margaret had other things on her mind.

'I couldn't do anything for her – she wouldn't even have a drink. It's always, "I'll wait until Deric comes home." She took seven pills with one tiny sip of orange. I know what it was. I told her she could drink all she wanted – I would take her to the toilet – I didn't mind, but no, she'd wait until you came home.'

Whenever I left for the day I would leave a tumbler of fresh orange on the bedside table. When I returned it would be virtually untouched.

To have to be helped to the toilet was Diana's idea of hell. What was the point in having your hair done, in painting your nails and wearing sexy nightdresses if you had to be helped to the toilet? How could any man fancy a woman he had to take to the toilet?

In the early days I would hear her crying with

shame as I waited outside the door to take her back to bed. Now she even had to be lowered down on to the seat.

But, over the years, I had convinced her that if there was anything I fancied in life, it was a woman that I could take to the toilet. She knew now that it made no difference – but still she preferred to keep it in the family.

Margaret went on: 'We talked for a long time.' She hesitated and then – 'Would Diana have any Soneryl? *I* haven't dispensed any for her.'

'My mother has Soneryl – or rather she did. They won't let her have sleeping tablets any more. . . . Why?'

'She asked me how many it would take – you know, to end it all. I wouldn't tell her, but she said she was sure she had enough.'

It didn't surprise me. We had talked about this – about the future. We had watched *Whose Life Is It Anyway?* on video, and Diana had wanted to know if I would help her finish it if life became too unbearable. 'I might not be able to pick up a pill in a year or so,' she had said.

Life doesn't prepare you for decisions like that – you can't go to night classes. Perhaps I would, but so far I had hedged my bets.

'She has three caches hidden,' Margaret told me. 'One in the kitchen, two in the bedroom. She said you wouldn't be able to find them.'

My mother certainly seemed to have cornered the

Soneryl market. Sixty a month over the past five years meant that some three thousand six hundred had passed through her hands, and not one had passed her own lips. I wondered how many Diana had.

'Thanks, Margaret – thanks for telling me.'

'Is there anything I can do?'

'Yes.'

'What's that?'

'If it's all right with you, I'd like to take my pants off.'

The night went on and on, as though tomorrow had been cancelled. Diana was exhausted now as her left hand began to follow suit – the right arm was on hold for the moment. Sometimes the virus played with her – cat and mouse. Once it had moved in so rapidly that we hadn't had time to remove Fred's plaster casts, and they had split and cracked like bridges caught in an earthquake.

The fingers of her left hand were biting into her palm, but that was as far as they would go. The left hand was nowhere near as professional as the right, and her toes were pathetic. They quivered slightly and, for an hour or so, they slowly twisted in on themselves, but they hadn't the stamina.

'Let me look,' asked Diana, and I rolled back the covers at the foot of the bed and then lifted her upright. She watched her toes as they twitched aimlessly.

140

'You're pathetic,' she shouted at them. 'Come on – shape up.'

She lay back on the pillows and the toes, embarrassed and confused, gave up and sulked.

Diana's digestive system had gone haywire over the past year and so I fed her bread and milk from a small spoon, trying not to look at the dish in my hand. The bread was no problem and neither was the milk, but once they had blended into a creamy modge it turned my stomach over. I had learned to simmer and dispense it blindfold.

'You're pushing it up my nose.'

'Sorry.'

We lay together and waited. I couldn't massage her arm because it was too painful, and so we waited for the next move.

'Where have you hidden the Soneryl?'

'Margaret told you.'

'You once asked me to help you – if it came to that.'

'Would you?'

'Probably.'

'Good.'

'I'd need to know where it was.'

'If it comes to that – I'll tell you.'

The virus returned with the early light and gripped Diana's arm in its teeth. First the back of her hand was forced hard up against her shoulder, and then the arm rolled remorselessly in on itself until her elbow was pressed against her ear.

The arm was locked solid and the pain excruciating. The first time it happened we had tried to break its hold – now we knew better. Sitting up, Diana rocked to and fro, side to side, swaying to a non-stop rhythm, and I brought hot towels and covered the arm. It had no effect whatsoever, but it made me feel useful and kept me busy.

She swayed and rocked for six hours, until midday, and then suddenly announced: 'It's going.'

The arm began to relax and unfold gradually until it was almost straight again – only the fingers told the story, more emaciated than before and still tightly clawed. We should have to work on them for a week or so, and then Fred would rebuild her.

I held her close and she began to cry – no need to be brave any more, it was all over for a time. Then the phone rang.

'I don't want to talk to anybody.'

I picked up the receiver. 'Hullo, Margaret.'

'I'll talk to her.'

I held the phone to her head on the pillow.

'No, no, really – I'm fine.'

10

It had been two weeks now since the attack and still Diana lay on her back in bed, her arms by her side, eyes lifeless, her voice faint and thin, her nose peeping over the sheets. Under the sheets were three hot water bottles – one under each leg and the third sitting up on her chest. Her feet were ice-cold, and this icing crept up her left leg to the biopsy scar on her thigh. Her hands were cold and she shivered, and I sat beside her and wiped the sweat from her forehead.

None of it made any sense. We could understand the doctor's confusion. We had to hold back when asked to describe the symptoms.

'I'll make a list,' Diana would say prior to a consultation. Then as she turned to the top of page three she would screw the paper into a ball. 'I think I'll play it by ear.'

It was too rich a diet for them – it gave them indigestion. At first they would nod wisely and then, as the symptoms piled up, they would gag at this feast of information. And then they would throw up – at least their hands in exasperation.

'We like to do our own tests – we'll start from scratch, shall we?'

*

Eating burned up too much energy and so it was kept down to a minimum – cereals, fruit and the dreaded bread and milk. The curtains would be closed as the light hurt her eyes, and my company was rationed on request.

'You go down now – watch the television.'

In the early days I hadn't understood. 'No – I'm all right. I'm quite happy here – nothing I want to watch, anyway.'

Eventually she pushed the message through to me. 'For Christ's sake, can't you see? If you're here I have to make an effort.'

I almost had the balance right now. No more, 'For Christ's sake . . . .' Just a quiet, 'Don't hover' every now and then. It was an improvement. Every hospital visitor should be handed, upon arrival, a card emblazoned with the legend: 'Don't hover.'

The breakthrough came as Sally arrived home for the weekend. Diana's arms appeared above the sheets and Sally and I celebrated in the kitchen with red wine and fish fingers. As the crocus heralds the first flush of spring, so Diana's arms, sunning themselves on the counterpane, heralded the second stage of her recovery. We looked forward to stage three when she would be propped up with pillows at her head and arms and, with the television remote control at her fingertips, ready to zap Mavis Nicholson if she went on a bit.

I was going to keep an eye on Sally this trip. It

144

was after her previous visit that it had gone missing. I always put it back where it belonged, Diana couldn't possibly have taken it, and Nick wouldn't touch it with a bargepole. There was only one other suspect and that was Sally – but you don't like to think that your daughter would steal a jar of Marmite.

I would never even have suspected her, but Diana had said, 'It was probably Sally.'

'Sally?'

'She must have taken it back with her.'

I couldn't believe it. 'She wouldn't just take it – she'd ask.'

'And what would you say if she asked?'

'I'd tell her to take it.'

'There you are, then.'

I had muttered something about it being the principle of the thing. Minutes before I had buttered two slices of bread, ready to be cut up into soldiers and lightly smeared with Marmite.

'I'll have apricot jam instead,' said Diana.

I had found the jam skulking at the back of the shelf, hiding behind the jar of prune puree that we seemed to have had since I was a lad. I could remember buying it. It was just before closing time and I could sense that the assistant wanted to be away. I rattled off the items on the list.

'Prawns,' I shouted.

'Prunes,' she repeated – and prunes I got.

We never ate prunes, which of course was why

the jar was still there. I kept meaning to throw it away at stocktaking every year, but it seemed such a waste.

Usually the jam was at the front, and when I opened it I found it to be less than half full. I had taken it upstairs to show Diana.

'I'm sure this was a virgin jar at the weekend.'

'Be Sally again,' Diana had nodded.

'You mean she's taken half of a jar of jam – what does she do, fill her handbag?'

Diana had then explained Sally's *modus operandi*. In her large canvas bag she had a dozen or so little plastic containers nestling neatly inside one another. During the weekend she would fill them – twenty or thirty teabags in this one, instant coffee in that. Here a little chutney, there a portion of Danish Blue. The odd jar of Marmite didn't need a container, but salad cream, sliced peaches and pineapple chunks travelled far better if cocooned in plastic.

'It's a spartan life – living in a bedsit,' Diana had told me. 'She needs a few luxuries.'

'But she only has to ask,' I had insisted. 'There's no need for her to smuggle the stuff out.'

'She likes to be independent – she doesn't want us to think she can't manage.'

Armed with this knowledge, it was fascinating to watch Sally in action. She stocked up on enough baths to last her a month, and after one of them she appeared in my office draped in a towel.

'Be a love and rub some of this on my back.'

She handed me Diana's body lotion and I dobbed a blob on to the palm of my hand and began rubbing. After about ten minutes I had very soft hands, but none of it was going into Sally's back. All I was doing was moving the lotion about.

'It's not going in.'

'Never mind,' she said, rising from the stool. 'I must be full – that's the fourth lot. I'll have a sunbed and wait for it to soak in.'

I rushed into the bedroom to tell Diana.

'She's smuggling out body lotion in her skin,' I told her. 'She must weigh a couple of pounds more than when she arrived.'

'That's clever.' Diana was impressed. 'She's also had seven goes on the sunbed.'

'She's on there now.'

'Eight,' said Diana.

Over the weekend it was a pleasure to watch a master kleptomaniac in action. A squirrel could only have sat back and watched in admiration.

I opened my wardrobe door to find three pairs of trousers on one hanger. Two coathangers gone walkabout – I wondered how she would fit them into her little plastic containers.

'Do you have any freezer bags?' asked Sally.

'How many do you want?'

'Half a dozen?'

She filled one with washing powder and another with flour. The others took raisins, sultanas and self-raising flour, while the sixth, to my amazement, was bloated with yoghurt. She must have run out of little plastic containers.

I seriously thought about setting up a red exit at the front door and a green 'Nothing to declare' exit at the back.

When the time came for her departure, she cuddled her mum whilst I carried her bag out to the car. It would have been easier to carry the car in to her bag.

She found me recovering in the kitchen. 'Are you all right?'

'I think I've just ruptured myself carrying your bag.'

'There's a knack to it,' she informed me as she shuffled two Elastoplast, a strip of aspirins and an elastic bandage out of the medicine chest and into her handbag.

On the way to the station I went through my usual routine.

'Are you all right for money?'

'Yes, thank you.'

'Are you sure?'

'Positive.'

'You don't want to be without.'

'I'm fine.'

'You can have a tenner if you want.'

'Dad,' she said firmly. 'I'm all right – you've got to realize that I'm independent now.'

I watched as the train pulled out of the station, and felt my groin quiver from the effort of heaving her bag into the carriage – I wish she had taught me the knack. But I smiled at the thought of my lovely independent daughter restocking her own little shelf in that antique fridge with her ill-gotten gains. It was going to take all night to unload that lot and I wondered what she would say when she found the tin of prune puree. I thought that would be a nice suprise.

The Maudsley Hospital in London had been very good about our cancelling Diana's appointment. 'Just ring when she's ready to come.'

I rang and fixed it for her to go in on the Wednesday, and began mentally reshuffling my week.

'I think I'll go by myself this time – on the train.'

I knew better than to argue at this early stage. She had made one or two trips by rail on her own, and it was an adventure that she relished. It scared the life out of me, but it gave her a taste of the independence she had once taken for granted.

To the average commuter the image of British Rail may come limping in a bad third behind toothache and dysentery, but I have no complaints about their handling of the disabled – emotionally or physically. A porter would meet us at the station and take over the wheelchair, trundling her across the rails to the far platform. The guard would have been alerted and a seat reserved. From the moment we passed through the barrier, I would become surplus to requirements. The guard would see that tea and sandwiches were brought to her, and at her destination another porter would be waiting to take over and whisk her through to the taxi rank. Never once a condescending word, and never once was the proffered tip accepted.

Even the taxi drivers came up trumps. Now and then page three of the *Sun* would prove magnetic and shield eyes that had already glimpsed the approaching wheelchair in a wing mirror, but there was always a driver willing to help the porter lift Diana, a buttock each, into the back of the cab. On her previous trip to the Maudsley the taxi driver had wheeled her right up to the reception desk before planting a kiss on her cheek and turning to leave.

'Wait! I haven't paid you yet.'

'Shut up or I'll let your tyres down.'

The anticipation of the trip would begin to flower as she settled in her seat with Dick Francis on her knee, and then it would burst into full bloom as my anxious little face and waving hand disappeared into the distance. She would sink into the sheer luxury of actually going somewhere without that accompanying face which, day after day, night after night, stood guard outside the toilet, winced as she was lowered into the bath, and continually searched her own face for the pain she tried so hard to hide.

On the train there would be new faces. Some would be hard and some uncertain, but many would smile, like the student with the green hair who still wrote every month, and with luck Dick Francis would remain a virgin to be deflowered later that night in the hospital ward.

She would miss me – but not yet. Those passengers who tumbled on to the train at later stations wouldn't see the wheelchair hidden away amongst the suitcases. She might get chatted up – she missed that. The plastered hands could be explained away as some dreadful accident, perhaps whilst scuba diving. It would add to the mystery.

Once in bed she had said: 'Do you realize – I couldn't have an affair even if I wanted to?'

'I could drive you there.'

'It wouldn't be the same.'

The train would be an adventure and she would log each incident as it happened, ready to pour it all out when next she saw that anxious face searching for her in the ward.

But now wasn't the time for adventures. She wasn't well enough, and the blackouts were coming thick and fast. Diana would have to make the decision – it's easy to put your foot down when your partner's legs don't work, but her brain worked well enough and the freedom to decide for herself was one of the few luxuries she had left.

Excited, she made all the arrangements with British Rail and planned the build-up meticulously. Two days of total rest with no visitors and no stress – on the Tuesday, little food or drink so as to avoid that rocking toilet on the train and, four hours before take-off, a well-researched cocktail of pain killers. It would work, it was just a case of mind over matter – if you wanted something badly enough you made it happen.

On the Tuesday night, as I packed her case, Diana sat up in bed and chatted incessantly.

'Are you sure you'll be all right?' she asked.

'I'll be fine.'

'You won't worry about me?'

'No – honest.'

'I'll be all right.'

'I know you will.' I intended to be in the next carriage disguised as a luggage rack or a sliding door or something. I had squared the matter with my conscience – if she didn't know I was there it wouldn't spoil her day, but I *would* be there. I was quite looking forward to the 'Follow that cab' stage in London.

'Well, you *look* worried.'

'No, I'm not – really.' Or I wouldn't be as soon as I had ironed out the problem of waving goodbye from the platform whilst sitting in the next carriage. I was working on a half-baked plan that involved using Nick as a diversion – it superseded the notion of hiring a Ferrari and beating the train to Leicester.

'I'm very capable.'

'I know you are.'

'Just a bit nervous.'

'That's understandable.' Could I see a crack

appearing in that brick-lined resolve? I carefully laid six pairs of tiny briefs in the case alongside the black basque. Not many women pack a black basque for the hospital – it was good to be married to an optimist.

'I suppose, if I had a blackout, it wouldn't really be fair on the other passengers.'

'That's a point, I suppose.' Yup! It was a little crack.

'But to hell with it. I've got to think about myself – they'll just have to put up with it.'

'That's the spirit.' Sod it!

I rounded up the tackle from the bathroom, leaving her toothbrush and make-up by the mirror for the morning. Towels! I always forgot towels. There, that was everything.

'Have you packed a flannel?'

'No.'

Later that night we sat in bed as Jim Rockford chatted to a stubby brunette outside the DA's office. Suddenly a bullet whistled past his ear, thudding into the door frame. Grabbing the girl, Jim ducked and weaved through the traffic. But the girl slowed him down and then another shot brought her to her knees. Jim bent over her, the blood oozing through her jacket, soaking his palm. Then darkness came as a rifle butt smashed against his skull.

'That's what I miss,' said Diana.

'Being beaten up?'

'Running across a road.'

So did I. Holding her hand and running across a road laughing, dodging the buses. With a wheelchair one has to wait on the pavement until it is safe. Being safe kills the free spirit inside you and turns you old before your time.

'Will you miss going down to London?'

'How do you mean?'

'Going round Foyle's and places after you've taken me to the hospital.'

'No.'

'Are you sure?' I glimpsed the crack once more.

'Well – no, not really. I've plenty to do here.'

'Come with me.'

'No. You'd rather try it alone.'

'I don't really feel well enough.'

I put my arm around her and gave her the last slice of the chocolate orange.

'All right, love – thank you.'

'I can always come back on my own when they let me out.'

11

The train was half empty, and we found two window seats at a table which we shared with a lady from Sheffield. She was an expert on the price of vegetables, especially sprouts, and later on we were joined by a gentleman from Leicester who wanted to bring back hanging. The rhythm of his argument faltered slightly just twice as I caught Diana's head inches above the table, but the sprout woman carried on bravely as she began to weave the noble turnip into the conversation.

Then the arm began to twist. First, clawlike, it threatened the hangman across the table, and then the hand turned over on to its back and the fingers began to close. Quickly I ripped away the Velcro from the plaster as the wire struts bent and the sprout woman, mouth open but mercifully silent for the moment, watched as the fingers bit into the palm and the knuckles lay flat against the wrist.

'Well – it's a cup of tea for me,' she declared when at last she found words.

'I'll join you,' sang the hangman with mock gaiety as he scrambled sideways from his seat.

As they disappeared towards the end of the carriage Diana began to sob silently, and I massaged her upper arm in the forlorn hope that it might just help.

I saw the sprout woman turn at the door and then clump back to stand over me. She cleared her throat and I looked up.

'Would you mind keeping an eye on our things?'

Diana gave a cry as her arm bent again.

'Only you can't trust anyone, can you?'

At other tables the passengers concentrated even harder on their crosswords and some slept on, occasionally opening one eye to monitor the drama across the aisle.

We stayed on the train for half an hour or so after it pulled into St Pancras. Cleaners cleaned around us, dropping cardboards cups into sacks. The guard, who had suspected initially that we were into some heavy necking, first threatened us with the police and then offered to send for an ambulance.

'We can manage – we just need a little time.'

'Tha' can have as long as tha' needs.'

'How long before it pulls out?'

'Dun't matter if it's late off – won't be first time.'

At the Maudsley I talked to the sister in her office as Diana was undressed and put to bed. She listened intently to my potted version of Diana's history for the first five seconds, and then her eyes were off through the glass on an inspection of the ward.

'Don't worry. We'll look after her. Now if you'll excuse me.'

I always found it difficult to take on the doctors and nurses. I could use words as they used a scalpel, cutting to the bone, but then I would be gone and Diana would remain – 'that woman with the awkward husband'.

She was too exhausted to talk at length, her eyes too heavy to focus.

'You go – I can manage.'

'I'll stay overnight, bed and breakfast somewhere and . . . .'

A nurse clattered over to the bedside, her sensible shoes rattling the senses, and a dozen glasses of orange juice trembled at her coming.

There is one in every hospital. They are schooled in the art of pillow thumping, mattress punching and talking very loudly and brightly when in the presence of husbands. This, they are told, is reassuring, and they learn to thump their pillows and punch their mattresses whilst at the same time smiling broadly at the dummy sitting in the chair by the bed.

'Come on, then. Let's sit up.'

'You can – I'm going to sleep.'

'You can sleep later. The doctor's coming to see you.'

'No.'

157

'Now we're not going to be awkward, are we?'

'I'm not, I'm going to sleep.'

'She needs to sleep,' I butted in. 'She's exhausted.'

I could see the sister approaching to add her considerable weight to the argument, and I braced myself ready for battle. She stroked Diana's forehead gently.

'I think we'll let Mrs Longden sleep, nurse. Mr Polkey won't want to see her until the morning.'

I could have kissed her, but she wouldn't have noticed. Those eyes slid past me to the bed in the far corner, and she was off down the ward to offer comfort.

So I kissed Diana instead and left for home. She was in good hands.

Outside my mother's house a bright yellow dustbin lorry chewed noisily on its cud as the driver climbed down to join his mate. Together they leaned against the wheel and waited.

I locked the car and walked towards them.

'Watch this,' he ordered, nodding towards the house.

The far trellis gate opened and my mother sailed up the path. I waved, but she didn't wave back. She was somewhat handicapped by the black plastic dustbin slung across her shoulders. The dustman walking behind her waved – but then he wasn't carrying anything.

'You shouldn't be carrying that,' I shouted.

'That's what I keep telling her,' the dustman agreed.

My mother stopped and turned, the dustbin still high on her shoulders. 'I'm not letting him carry it – he ruptured himself.'

'That was years ago,' muttered the dustman miserably. 'Four years ago.'

My mother continued her march up the path. 'You tell him how it can go again just like that – go on, you tell him.'

'It can go again – just like that,' I told the dustman.

'My husband,' said my mother, 'his father – ruptured himself and all he did was cough.'

Now I had to admit that was true. My father did rupture himself and all he did was cough.

'He was picking up a three hundredweight bag of peat at the same time,' I reminded her.

'All the more reason why *he* shouldn't lift dustbins,' declared my mother, and for the first time since the conversation began I could see a glimmer of logic shining through.

The dustman squirmed as his mates grinned at him over the wall.

'I have to pick up dustbins,' he muttered. 'I'm a dustbin man.'

'Just so long as you don't rupture yourself picking up *my* dustbin,' said my mother, and then all four of us jumped on her as she attempted to hurl the entire contents of the bin deep into the bowels of the cart.

★

Whisky poked his head nervously round the kitchen door as I carried the empty bin back in the yard. He rarely ventured out during the winter months, as my mother began to feed the birds again and this year a particularly butch robin was making his life a misery. Her garden is a sort of ornithological Little Chef and the birds come from miles around. She gets all the business simply because she goes to more trouble than her neighbours – she doesn't merely chuck a few stale slices of bread on to the lawn, she believes that even your most yobbo sparrow likes things nice.

A large bag of assorted nuts hangs from the cherry tree as a starter, and there is always fresh water in the bird bath so that fastidious diners can rinse their beaks before and after. Unfortunately some of the more uncouth customers rinsed rather more than their beaks before dining. The sparrows were in there up to their wingpits, whistling obscenities at the blue tit who was merely mopping the corner of his beak on the edge.

'They like the crusts cut off,' she told me as she attacked the sliced loaf with the bread knife. 'Birds don't have all that many teeth, you know.' Then she poured a trickle of warm milk over the cubes so that, I imagine, the poor little old-age pensioner birds, who had no teeth at all, could enjoy a trouble-free nibble.

She spread the bread upon a tin tray and sprinkled it with an enormous quantity of All Bran. 'They need the roughage,' she said in answer to my unasked question, and Whisky gave me a knowing look. Through the window the trees were coated with a white emulsion which now covered the old-fashioned pink of the raspberry season – the last thing the birds seemed to need was roughage.

She chucked a handful of currants over the offering and, just as I thought she might pipe it with icing, she picked up the tray and made for the kitchen door.

The noise was horrendous – straight from the Hitchcock film. There were sparrows, of course, hundreds of them competing with blackbirds, thrushes, tits – blue and otherwise – doves by the drove and ponderous pigeons, and they welcomed my mother as though she were the Ayatollah Khomeini come to lead them in prayer.

She moved majestically down the path broad-casting the bread to the farmost corners of the lawn, and some of the smaller sparrows were slightly con-cussed as they were clobbered on the head by a well-soaked chunk of Mother's Pride.

By the time she had returned, the lawn had been picked clean and the flock had taken off like a bomber squadron for a sweet course of rotting crab apples at number 103.

Whisky crept out of his breadbin bunker to stare at the few little Oliver Twists begging for seconds at the window, and my mother and I moved into the lounge for a well-earned coffee, a digestive biscuit and a nice long chat.

'How was Diana when you left her?'

Nervous, apprehensive, frightened, lonely, defiant – all those things and many more. Life in a hospital is one big confidence trick – a performance. Doctors playing Kildare, bantering nurses with hearts of gold. Orderlies playing the fool and patients ancient and modern, fragile and brave, acting out a part they have never rehearsed.

'You should have stayed with her.'

No. When she was far away and I couldn't be there at visiting time each day, it was better if I left her to it. She could sink into the life of the ward and pretend that nothing else existed outside. She could get on with it – get it over. After a visit from me she had to start again from scratch. I brought with me all that she was missing.

'So you won't be going down?'

Yes. The theory was one thing – in practice I missed her dreadfully, and I needed a shot of that half smile that would greet me as I walked in the ward. The smile that told me, 'I knew you would come.' I needed to know – to see for myself, to touch her. Perhaps it was better to take the pain of parting once again, rather than the Valium of pretence. In short – selfishly, I needed to go and see her, so that she could visit me.

'Perhaps they'll find something this time.'

And perhaps not. Mr Polkey had told us that he would start from scratch. A myelogram and other tests – but he had tried before and he had that air about him. An air of pale confidence that I had seen so many times before, worn by doctors in Sheffield, Derby and London and by that motor mechanic in Chesterfield as he bent under the bonnet of my old Audi.

'Anyway – what have you been doing with yourself lately?'

Yes, let's change the subject. I looked at my watch.

'I'm on "Woman's Hour" any minute.'

'Oh!'

She had listened to my first broadcast many years ago, and since then I had occasionally let her know when I was on again. I always met with the same response: 'Well, I've heard you before.' She seemed to think I repeated the same material over and over again – perhaps she was right. But this time she wasn't going to get away with it. I switched on the radio and fiddled until I heard Sue McGregor talking to Margaret Drabble. I was in good company – my mother had heard of neither of them.

Ms Drabble told us that she used 'Woman's Hour' as a barometer of public taste. Sue McGregor had an ace up her sleeve.

'Well, just stay for a moment and listen to Deric Longden, Margaret.'

I sneaked a glance at my mother to see if she was impressed. She was halfway under the settee after Whisky's ping-pong ball.

'Deric might help you change your mind.'

I mentioned AIDS, full frontals and naked bodies in the first half minute, and then launched into a piece about rams and ewes making wild passionate love. Quite how I managed it I can't remember.

My mother sat, cat on her knee, staring at the radio as though it were a television set. I stared at the ceiling.

I finished – Sue McGregor introduced the serial and my mother stared at the cat.

The silence is the worst thing. It's wonderful if someone says, 'That was terrific – that was great!' If they tell you that it wasn't perhaps one of your best efforts – well, I can cope with that. But the silence . . . .

She broke the silence. 'Another cup of coffee?'

We walked through to the kitchen. I was damned if I was going to ask her what she thought.

'What did you think?'

She measured a spoonful of coffee into the mug, flicked the switch on the kettle and turned to face me.

'I do wish your father had let me send you for elocution lessons.'

The Ocean Pie was in the oven – 180 degrees for twenty minutes, it said on the packet. As long as it told me what to do on the box, I could cook it. Ocean Pie, Cumberland Pie, Cod Mornay, Duckling à l'Orange. We lived well, but at the mercy of Marks & Spencer's. Once I had tried broccoli, but when I tipped it out of the carrier bag I could see it was simply wrapped in clingfilm. I searched the packet for instructions – nothing, so I stuck it in a vase on the mantelpiece.

Twenty minutes. What was it Margaret had said? 'She has three caches hidden. One in the kitchen, two in the bedroom. She said you would never find them.' Twenty minutes. Where would you hide a small packet of Soneryl in a small kitchen? I began in the larder, top shelf first, and worked my way down, wiping clean the jars and containers until the shelves sparkled with a lemon-scented freshness. Sultana and raisin jars were thoroughly shaken and stirred, and the flour bins raked with a fork. Soon the whole larder gleamed but, apart from a lonely and somewhat dispirited iced bun lodged behind the gas meter, nothing had been unearthed.

I added two individual fruit pies to the oven and decanted a packet of frozen peas into a pan. When I first took over the cooking we had lived on fish fingers and frozen peas until the kids had complained of frostbite. Nowadays our diet had become far more sophisticated. We no longer existed on such peasant fare – we had petits pois, which are very much like frozen peas, but they've been killed while they were still pups.

I prised the lid from a drum of custard and poured milk into a saucepan. I was especially proud of my custard. In the early days it had poured like yellow milk – then someone taught me how to 'boil it back'. Now I made it so thick I had to slice it.

I pushed my chair from the table. 'Apple pie and custard?'

'Lovely.' Nick shifted behind his paper. 'You going down to the hospital this weekend?'

'Yes.'

'I'll be on my own, then.'

For about five minutes, I thought, as I brought two miserable, overcooked pies out of the oven. I had some sliced apple in reserve, but it had gone off. Why does sliced apple go rusty?

I cut the custard down the middle, slipped the spatula under a generous half, and with my left hand picked up a plate that had baked in the oven for fifteen minutes at 180 degrees. The result was electrifying. The solid block of custard shot over my right shoulder and bounced three times across the floor, like Barnes Wallis's bomb, before slamming against the kitchen door.

As I plunged my hand into cold water, I watched the custard slide gently down the door and then squat awkwardly on the carpet tiles. On my hands and knees I examined the problem and then, with the spatula, prised the carpet tile away from its mates and carried it ceremoniously over to the draining board, dropping the nervous yellow lump on to Nick's apple pie. After a quick scrub down the tile was back in place and I was back at the table. Nick had been plotting.

'I'll stay in on Saturday night. Then you can ring me – tell me how Mum is.'

'You don't have to do that.'

'I'd like to know.' He toyed with his pie. 'Jo might like to keep me company – and Ian and Rob Hunt and Jez York.'

'You could get a few beers in.'

'That's a thought.' He dug a spoon into his dish and examined it closely. 'There's all hairs on my custard.'

'It's bran – I'm trying to keep you regular.'

'Oh,' he tasted a sample and then dug in heartily. 'Nice – very nice. Makes all the difference.'

As Nick washed up I emptied the plate cupboard looking for the Soneryl. Then I pulled out the knife drawer and began sifting through the spare cork-screw area at the back.

'What are you looking for?'

'Nothing.'

'Hope you find it.'

I slid the drawer back into place and moved on to teatowels and sundry linen.

'I've lost some pills – they're in the kitchen somewhere.'

'Are they in a bottle?'

'Yes – have you seen it?'

'No.'

'They could be in a drum – or a polythene bag.'

'You're not sure?'

I didn't like being evasive – I could lie my head off over custard – but this was important. Even so. . . .

'Your mum's mislaid them.'

Nick was drying his hands. 'Pink pills – in a polythene bag?'

'Yes.'

He bent down and pulled the shoe-cleaning kit from under the sink. Folding back a duster, he produced a Cherry Blossom boot polish tin and handed it to me.

I flirted off the lid. The inside had been thoroughly wiped clean and the pink pills shone through the Midland Bank change-bag, 'Acceptable contents, £5 –10p'.

I spilled the sleeping tablets on to a plate and counted them – twenty-seven.

Nick picked one up and examined it. 'How many would it take?'

'About eight – how did you know they were there?'

'The Pavilion party – I was going to black up.'

We were quiet as I slipped them back in the bag, resealed the tin and placed the whole works back where we had found it.

I wanted to swill the tablets down the sink – but did I have the right? It was her life, and I couldn't just take it over. God knows how long it had taken

her to clean out the tin. I could think about this later
– I had time.

'She told Margaret that she'd hidden them where
we'd never find them.'

Nick looked down first at my shoes and then at
his own. 'Not daft, is she?'

12

The day really took off with a bewildering phone call. Having already coped with a seven-thirty blast from my mother – her opening salvo being, 'Whatever happened to Edgar Lustgarten?' – I should have been prepared for anything, but the lady from Chester left me speechless. She was Madam Secretary and I was booked to speak at her club on the 14th. She was just checking.

'We have a microphone if you need one.'

'About how many in the audience?'

'A hundred – hundred and twenty.'

'I think I can manage without.'

She was very efficient. I once asked a luncheon club secretary if she would mind providing a carafe for me, and I arrived to find a five-foot-tall, solid oak lectern standing on the stage. Trumpet-blowing cherubs clambered up its sides and an enormous golden eagle straddled the peak. She had dragged it single-handed from the local church.

After twenty minutes or so I needed a sip of water, and so I bent and whispered.

'Where's the carafe?'

'That's it,' she said, prodding a cherub.

'That's a lectern.'

'Damn it – I always get them mixed up.'

But the lady from Chester was in a different class altogether. A timetable and route map were to be dispatched by the next post – and then she dropped her bombshell. She hesitated for a moment and asked, 'Is that the voice you'll be using when you speak?'

It threw me completely. What could I say? 'Well, not if it doesn't suit – I have a box here under my desk containing several other voices. How about this one?' Instead I answered meekly: 'Er – yes.'

'Oh, well.' She seemed resigned. 'I suppose it will be all right.'

I could feel a small but beautifully marked complex crouching on my left shoulder ready to spring, fully grown, the moment I arrived in Chester.

I had arranged to drive to BBC Radio Derby – go live on their 'Line Up' programme, record a piece down the wire for Radio Nottingham's 'The Sporting Week' and then, leaving the car, catch the train to London.

Lesley, the programme secretary at Derby, poured me a coffee and stirred it gently with her biro so as not to disturb the penicillin incubating in the bottom of the mug. Ashley Franklin, the producer, told me that next week the programme would be broadcast live from the new public lavatories in Heanor. Now I knew why I went through this every week – it wasn't the money, it was the glamour. On the other side of the glass Graham Knight, the presenter, read out a listener's letter written on House of Commons toilet paper, and when I joined him we discussed which way you should hang a toilet roll. Should the next available sheet hang towards the wall or away from it?

On a cue from Graham I launched into a six-minute solo on toilet paper in general:

'This country is in danger of being overrun by pink toilet rolls – I don't mean that gentle pastel pink designed to melt into the background of a rose-hued bathroom. The newcomers are a harsher, acne-flushed shade of pink that seems to have been achieved by dropping the roll into a toilet and then drying it slowly over a peat fire for a fortnight.

'You can see them everywhere – they breed in dump bins just inside the door of any second-string chemist and then make their way, during the hours of darkness, into the toilets of transport cafés and cinemas.

'When I made my first sighting I assumed that it was from a batch that had gone wrong and was being sold off cheap. But now they are everywhere – the little perforations are purely for decoration, the sheets rip off at random and the whole effect suggests a toilet roll that has given up on life and let itself go to rack and ruin.

'Very soon we shall see these toilet rolls squatting in alleys and drinking meths straight from the bottle. The police will have to be called to move them on, and it won't be safe for decent citizens to go out of the house after nightfall . . .'

And so on and so on, until Graham eased himself back behind the console and took over the reins once again. Sometimes I felt that my function, halfway through the three-hour programme, was simply to allow the presenter to go to the toilet.

'Thanks, Deric,' shouted Ashley as I made my way out of the studio. 'Don't ring us – we'll ring you.'

A phone rang in the control room and then there was a crash as it hit the floor.

'Shit,' a voice cried out. It seemed most appropriate.

Down in the news studio I spoke to Andy Knowles in Nottingham. I was particularly proud of the piece I was about to record. It had pace, wit and style. It was intelligent and thoughtful and I had handled it with an exceptionally light touch.

'The tape's rolling,' Andy told me, and I laid down this five-minute gem without a single fluff – my voice enhancing the quality of the script. I was feeling smug – Andy would be impressed.

'That it?' he wanted to know.

'Yes.'

'Talk to you next week, then,' and he was gone.

The bastard. If it wasn't for the fact that I was in love with his wife I'd never work for him again.

I tried to work on the train. A writer should be able to work anywhere – all he needs is a pad and a pencil whereas a vet, for instance, would be frowned upon by his fellow passengers if he laid out his instruments and attempted to castrate a small gerbil.

But a writer has this freedom – except that I can't work in company. I stared at the blank pad for an hour or so, and then settled for jotting down a few important questions that I needed to ask Diana. Questions such as:

'Can you eat cherry pie filling on its own?'

'Where are the nail scissors?'

'How do you stop the radio alarm going off at three in the morning?' and

'What do you do with rice?'

I opened the rather smart briefcase that Nick had given me for my birthday, tucked my notepad under a pair of pants and took out a cheese sandwich. A job well done.

Diana wasn't available for questioning. She had been moved to a smaller ward – so small it took some finding. Her bed was empty, but the sister put me in the picture.

'She's gone down for a myelogram.'

Diana had been apprehensive about the myelogram. This was to be her fourth, and it was an unpleasant business. A small amount of spinal fluid is drawn off, then a contrast medium, a sort of dye, is introduced, after which the spine is X-rayed. Most people suffer no ill effects whatsoever, but on each of the previous occasions Diana had been sick and suffered violent headaches afterwards – she could handle that, but after the first myelogram she knew what to expect and the anticipation was almost as bad as the test itself.

'Would you like to go down and wait for her to come out?'

'Yes, please.'

A small, wiry nurse was appointed my guide and off we set to find Diana.

'She's all right, your wife, isn't she?'

'I like her.'

'Have you seen her embroideries? Well, you will have, won't you – aren't they good? I don't know how she does it what with her hands – she's teaching me. She's given me one of her frames and some silks, but I'm not very artistic – I want to do a rabbit for my mum.'

I'm sure she was wearing running shoes, and I had a hell of a job keeping up with her.

'How has she been?'

'She was exhausted when she came in – we made her rest for two days. She needs lots of rest – she was knackered. I've seen lots of patients like Diana – they fight it and they shouldn't. I don't know what it is, but it's something that gets at them. It's no good fighting it.'

Her tongue continued to keep pace with her feet as we rattled down the corridors, but she made a lot of sense.

For some time now I'd had a nagging feeling that we had made mistakes in the early days. Diana had fought the exhaustion and battled on. We knew now from experience that rest, complete rest, was the only way to keep her on a even keel. Maybe, if she had taken it easy from the start, things might have been different – but often in hospital their only aim seemed to be to get her on her feet as quickly as possible and hand her over to the physiotherapist. I have every admiration for physiotherapists – but in Diana's case they seemed to have done more harm than good.

'She needs peace as well – she doesn't want shouting at. You don't shout at her, do you?'

'No.'

'I should hope not. She's cheered everybody up – she's been trying to cheer up the lady in the next bed, only she doesn't want to be cheered up. She likes being miserable, and she's been grumbling about Diana cheering her up, so Diana told her she was a miserable bugger and that made her miserable and so she's happy now.'

I thought that I followed that – I should enjoy meeting the lady in the next bed.

'It's just round this corner – Diana was very nervous when they took her down. They're always nervous when they've had a myelogram before – they know what it's like. You can't lie to 'em. Anyway, I'll see you later. She's in there.'

She indicated a pair of swing doors and I sat down in the antiseptic hallway and waited.

I seemed to have done so much waiting over the

past few years. Up to this point I had simply looked forward to seeing Diana again – but now, as I sat alone in this stark white hall, I began to feel very weary. I was losing weight – far too much weight. I had an ulcer and I could no longer eat properly. My face looked worn and haggard. Too many friends these days asked anxiously, 'Are you all right?' the minute they clapped eyes on me.

Financially I was being attacked on all sides, and I had been pulling the wagons into a circle for some time. I'd just about run out of wagons. I was tired out, I felt pathetic and I was thoroughly ashamed of myself. It's the emotional skirmishes that sap the energy. Whilst you are under fire the adrenalin keeps pumping, but I had just slept through five consecutive nights – no hot baths to administer, no pretending to be asleep with one ear cocked while Diana moaned in pain. Just five nights of deep, deep sleep, and in the morning I could be where I had said I would be – on time.

I'd even had a steak in the Berni – upstairs! I had leapt into the car and driven off – no tucking of legs in the passenger well, no stowing of wheelchairs in the boot. Just straight into first gear and off. The freedom to act without having to calculate the odds against is a joy that is never appreciated until it's been lost. I had tasted that freedom for a week, and I had enjoyed it and I felt as guilty as hell.

It's a guilt that all carers know well. You are hobbled by responsibilities – live life in the slow lane and watch old bangers flying past and you know you could leave them standing if only. . . . It's a guilt that the cared-for know also, and it hurts them far more.

'If it wasn't for me.'

'Don't be silly.'

It's a guilt that is rarely brought out into the light and it can fester in the shadows. The only antidote is love and that, thank God, I had in bucketsful.

The swing doors broke open and a trolley poked its nose out and then stopped. A pair of feet lay on the trolley – Diana's feet. I'd have known them anywhere, the right ankle slim and elegant, the left grown thick from disuse. The star of the movie and her best friend.

I half rose. Where was the rest of her? Then a commotion and shouted orders from behind the door. Then I knew – she was dead. I moved forward and the right leg kicked. The trolley burst out of the room and stopped again.

Diana writhed and twisted – her wrists crossed over her face covering her eyes. She banged her head again and again, hard against the side of the trolley. A nurse clamped her head and swung her on to her side. The body heaved, up and down, up and down – the right leg kicked, the back arched and a doctor shouted. The trolley moved on and up the corridor followed by a flurry of white coats. I stood and stared after it and watched as it turned the corner.

Not until the trolley had disappeared from sight

did any part of me work. My brain had taken it all in, but it wasn't giving orders.

By the time I reached the ward she had been shovelled into bed and under the blankets. Through a circle of white coats I could see the sister – she was holding Diana's hand and, at the same time, pressing a wet towel over her face, gently massaging her eyes and forehead with tender fingertips through the towel.

The blanket pulsed, but the movements were not as convulsive now and the shoulders under the white coats had relaxed. I forced myself to stand back and wait – no time for questions yet, let them get on with it.

The wiry little nurse spotted me and nudged a white coat – he turned and came over.

'What's happened?'

'I've no idea. She went into a convulsion – she isn't an epileptic, is she?'

'No.'

'I've never seen this before – we had to abort the myelogram. There could have been pressure on the brain – I'm not sure.'

They never did find out what had happened. Several theories were put forward, but none of them seemed to bear close examination. It was just another mystery to add to the string, and sometimes there are no answers to the questions – the old-timers know this and accept that it happens. The first-timers and once-in-a-life-timers often kick up a stink, but it's a waste of time and energy and Diana had little to waste.

For the next two days she lay in bed, her eyes shielded from the light and unable to move her head an inch either way without awakening the sickening pain behind her eyes. She had been sick until she could be sick no longer, and now we waited for the mists to clear.

For most of the two days I had tucked myself in by the bed, squatting on a chair which had been ergonomically designed to support the back, cushion the knees and drill little holes in the backside. I read softly to her, a letter from Sally, my column from the *Matlock News*, that piece for 'The Sporting Week' that Andy Knowles had dismissed with, 'Is that it?' Diana squeezed my hand and I bent my head to try and catch her words.

'No more.' Perhaps it wasn't as riveting as I had imagined. When she squeezed my hand again it was a signal for me to begin once more, and I moved into the safer area of local gossip.

Even though it hurt Diana to move her lips and the blessed chair was sucking in huge lumps from my backside, we somehow managed to communicate far more than did 'The miserable woman in the next bed' and her husband. His name was Derek, like mine – spelt differently, but then perhaps his father wasn't illiterate – and, when spoken aloud, just the same. He was a cost accountant and a saint. She had multiple sclerosis and was a martyr.

She was ill, there was no doubt about it, but she was also the centre of the universe and she complained about everything. Derek sat by her bed and watched her suffer. If he made a move to pick up a magazine she moaned and he would lay it down. If he looked away for a second she moaned and he would look back guiltily. His job was to sit there and play the part of the concerned husband – it wasn't a speaking part, it wasn't a walking-on part. He just had to sit there, and he did it beautifully.

Diana had fallen asleep and I needed a cigarette. Out in the corridor was a fire bucket full of sand in which I had played happily for hours over the past two days – I could keep an eye on Diana through the glass and smoke, and bury the evidence in the bucket. The contents were now ninety-eight per cent filter-tip, topped off with a two per cent crust of sand. If we had a fire it would be interesting.

I tapped Derek on the shoulder, 'Fancy a smoke?'

He shook his head wistfully.

'Come on – you'll be able to see her through the glass.'

He looked back at his wife and watched her nostrils flutter as she snored.

I tried again, 'Come on.'

He rose on tiptoe, and in a cowering crouch he followed me towards the door. Or maybe I misjudged him – perhaps he had piles.

He was halfway across the room when his wife felt a tug on the invisible cord that held him prisoner. Her weak, helpless voice caught up with him as he passed the fire extinguisher. It was a voice that whined with self-pity – it was a weapon she used like a blowpipe.

'Derrr-eeeek!'

It stopped him in his tracks. He smiled at me – a Stan Laurel smile – and then he turned and dipped back into his cage.

There are many men who, when faced with the prospect of looking after a crippled wife, can't take it and leave. More than you would ever imagine. I have always thought it shameful and have never been able to understand the shallowness of such men – and yet.

'Derrr-eeeek.'

If that pathetic wail were to shadow me twenty-four hours a day – then perhaps I would be on the first bus out of town.

I could do without the cigarette and I went back to talk to Derek – to show him that I understood, that perhaps he was stronger than I could ever be, but as I opened my mouth to speak he put his finger to his lips and shushed me.

I laid my hand on Diana's. She had seen nothing, yet heard it all, and she stroked her wrist against mine.

'Go and have a smoke . . . ,' she whispered.

'I don't need one.'

' . . . and a drink. . . . '

'I'm all right here.'

' . . . and screw one of the nurses.'

'Oh, all right then.'

My job was nowhere near as hard as Derek's. Had he brought it on himself, or had he little choice? I was just happy that I had the strength to carry on, and I knew exactly where that strength came from.

I have a theory about disablement. It changes the victim – but not as much as people think. The optimist remains an optimist, albeit with a flaky eye. The miserable sod who loses his left leg doesn't change – he simply becomes a miserable sod with one leg.

A couple of days later Diana was back to normal, whatever that was, and we decided to go over the wall for an hour or so.

As we left the Maudsley behind us and eased our way down Denmark Hill, I had ample opportunity to test the theory. It was as though we were taking part in a vintage wheelchair rally – half the population of SE5 seemed to be sitting down and the other half were pushing them towards Camberwell Green. We stared in wonder at the odd electric Porsche, admired the middle-range Volvos and mentally tooted our horn at the many mirror images of our own National Health Lada.

I can't explain the compulsion to stop and talk to fellow victims. Perhaps it just seems rude to pass in silence, but more often than not there is little to be found in common other than the fact that one can't walk and the other is in harness – it's rather like two mothers stopping to chat merely because the kids are wearing the same school blazer.

It's all a matter of levels. On the top floor the mothers find they have little to talk about whilst down below in the basement the kids meet, eyeball to eyeball, and loathe each other on sight. It's a bit like wife swopping – it's rare for all four to enjoy the experience. And yet you stop and talk, and never about the weather or the state of the nation.

'We can't go too far now – she's incontinent,' the tall man with the hairy nostrils told us, nodding down at the back of his wife's head. 'But I like her to have a breath of fresh air.'

His wife buried herself deeper into the wheelchair – trying to make herself invisible as yet another complete stranger was told what a burden she had become.

'It's her spinal cord, you see – it's gone. It affects the bladder, does that.'

Diana glared at him. She had a glare that could stun a buffalo at thirty paces, but his solid teak sensitivity was impenetrable and so she turned her attention to his victim with words of comfort.

But there was nobody in. The woman's spirit had first been bruised by pain and fear and finally battered to death by a man with hairy nostrils.

*

Like nannies in a nineteenth-century park we paraded further down the concrete strip to a zebra crossing where two other nannies waited. Their charges held hands across the wheels, and all four had that unnatural light in their eyes.

I pulled Diana up level on the starting grid and we nodded politely. A spare hand patted Diana's knee sympathetically.

'How long has it been, my dear?'

'Too long.'

'Never mind – it's God's will.'

'God's will!' echoed her companion, and then the traffic stopped and, cutting across our bows, they floated serenely across the road – eyes on full beam lighting the way.

'God's will be buggered,' Diana muttered as the traffic surged forwards, leaving us stranded.

'He got 'em across the road,' I told her as we waited for the next break. 'He parted the Cortinas.'

I've seen that light so many times and often wondered if it survives the night, after the curtains have been drawn. Or is it painted on each morning? Whatever – it helps them cope and good luck to them, but I don't think I want anything to do with a God like that.

We sat on a bench in Camberwell Green and ate ice cream and felt very old until we were joined by a couple who made us feel very young. He man-oeuvred the chair with difficulty until it butted up to

Diana's, and then he creaked down beside me on the bench.

'Where are they all coming from?' he wanted to know. 'Is it a rally or something?'

'I've no idea – I assumed they were all from the hospital.'

'I've never seen as many as this.' He tucked the tartan blanket tighter round his wife. 'I feel I ought to have decorated her up as a float.'

They were perhaps in their late seventies, she a heavyweight, he a flyweight, and they held hands as they talked.

'I was an engineer – up in Luton. We had a lovely house – I liked Luton.'

His wife leaned forward. 'With a little paddock and a goat called Maurice.'

He remembered fondly. 'Oh yes – Maurice. I'd forgotten Maurice.'

She went on. 'He had to give up work when I took ill. We're in sheltered housing now – it's all ramps and a warden.'

He came out of his reverie. 'I was bigger than she was then – hard to imagine, isn't it?'

'He worries about me, you see – it's just dropped off him, whereas I don't get any exercise, not stuck in this chair. I was seven stone when I married him.'

'Now I've got twice as much as I bargained for – not bad that, is it?'

As they talked they stole quick glances at one

another – touched each other as though each time might be the last time, and then held hands again.

'I don't know what I'd do without him – if I lost him, I don't know what I'd do.'

There was a real fear in her eyes, and he tucked and retucked the rug around her.

'Come on, then – let's have you home.'

They said their goodbyes and we watched them cross the pavement to their arthritic Hillman. The wheelchair footrests were flicked back with a practised hand, but it was becoming more than hard work for him to lift her from the chair.

I moved across to help, but he was ready for me.

'I can manage – thank you.'

And he did – just about. But the effort took it out of him and his wife looked wary as she trusted herself to his arms. The wheelchair was buried in the boot with the help of bumper and knees – no clean lifts nowadays. He paused, leaning on the car, before settling in the driving seat.

'Bye, then.'

We sat and watched as the car slowly pulled away. We were quiet long after it had disappeared, and then Diana said: 'That's my future.'

And mine, I thought.

'And yours,' she said.

187

13

'No more hospitals,' said Diana as the train pulled out of St Pancras and headed north. 'That's it – from now on we handle it on our own.'

The Maudsley had come up with nothing. We hadn't expected them to – we knew better than that – but it was always disappointing. A second myelogram had proved an ordeal for Diana, but it had shown nothing apart from the odd cyst on the spine.

'It must be a virus,' she declared, and the lady sitting opposite seemed to agree and nodded approvingly.

It had begun ten years ago with what we thought was Asian flu – and the doctor agreed, suggesting: 'Plenty of rest, plenty of liquid and some aspirin.' The fever had passed, but the fatigue had remained and with it the pain which had worked away at her arms and legs until they were weak and the exhaustion began to take over her life. An hour's rest would help, but within minutes she was back to square one and she tumbled through life as though she had missed a week's sleep – her memory was not as it was and, as her hands and feet grew colder, she would be bathed with perspiration.

'Have you tried alternative medicine?' asked the lady sitting opposite. 'It worked wonders for me.'

She was pale and uninteresting. When Diana was at her worst the colour would drain from her face, but the lady sitting opposite had a complexion that was white as a geisha and I tried to imagine what she must have looked like before alternative medicine had worked its wonders.

We received a lecture on faith healing and holistic medicine that was comprehensive, to say the least, and I was grateful that she wasn't able to illustrate it with slides. She left the train with us at Derby and completed her lecture in the car park. It was drizzling with rain and she sat sideways on the driver's seat whilst I tucked the wheelchair into the boot. Eventually I managed to prise her out of the car and we started out on the last lap home.

Diana pulled down the vanity mirror. 'Do I look as bad as she did?'

'Even I don't look as bad as she did.'

We drove in silence down the dual carriageway that passes for a town centre in Derby, and then Diana asked, 'Do you think there's anything in it?'

'I don't know – maybe.' We moved out into the suburbs. 'Do you remember that faith healer I interviewed?'

'I remember you were impressed with him.'

'He lives about a mile further on – why don't we try him?'

'When?'

189

'Now.'

'We can't just drop in like that – he'll have a waiting list.'

'If he has he'll tell us – we might be lucky. If we don't do it now, we'll never come back.'

She thought about it.

'It's just round this corner,' I told her.

'I don't think I even believe in it.'

'Next turn on the left.'

'Go on, then – let's give it a try,' and I turned into an avenue lined with trees and pulled up in front of the house.

A woman answered the door. She was sorry – her husband had a full appointment book.

'But I could see you – I've nothing until three.'

We left the wheelchair in the hall and she took us through to a drawing room. I manhandled Diana across the room until she was sitting in a low-back chair in the middle. The woman took a pendulum from around her neck and stood behind the chair.

'Just relax and ask me anything you like.' She laid her hand on Diana's neck and held the pendulum above her head.

'Did you meet your husband through faith healing?' Diana wanted to know.

'No – but he gets very busy and he taught me so that I could help out.'

That seemed very convenient. I could imagine a healer teaching a pupil because he sensed they had a

190

gift, but his wife so that she could help out? A little too handy for my liking.

She moved the pendulum down Diana's spine and it jumped and twisted. There was a silence that lasted some minutes, and then the woman replaced the stone around her neck and laid her hands on Diana's back. The silence thickened and we didn't break it with questions – it had a feel about it.

'There,' said the woman. 'You'll be much better in a day or two.'

'What did you do?'

'You had five discs out of place in your spine – I've put them back.'

Our hopes hit the floor with a thud. Diana slipped me a glance – she had been quite caught up in the magic.

'But I had a myelogram the day before yesterday – it showed that no discs were out of place.'

'Ah, well!' said the woman, 'you know what hospitals are like.'

I paid her, twelve pounds I think it was, and we drove home. We only mentioned the healer in passing – we quietly worked away separately at the same thought. It was too much of a disappointment to get angry about it. As hospital after hospital had failed to come up with a diagnosis we had kept fringe medicine in reserve – a dark horse to be gambled on when all else had failed. And now we had tried it and it had fallen at the first fence.

*

For a week or so we couldn't pick ourselves up – it was as though someone had died in the house. The love that flowed between us so naturally under the surface and brought with it an effortless supply of harmony, tenderness and passion seemed now to be visible. The little courtesies and pleasantries that love eases into position so guilelessly appeared now to be so obvious – as though performed by strangers. We were each wrapped up in our own thoughts – thoughts of the future – and for the first time ever we seemed to be living together, apart. The distance between us was illuminated by an unnatural politeness.

'Would another bath help?'

'It would, really – if it's not too much trouble.'

'No – not at all.'

I could have been a home help, drafted in because the usual one was off sick.

Since first we had met, the kindness and consideration we had shown to each other had sprung unannounced from a love that was never questioned – now we were having to work at it. I began to experience an eerie feeling – that whatever I was doing, I was standing over on the other side of the room watching myself do it – watching myself acting out a part. Sitting up in bed reading one night, I put down my book and touched her hand.

'I'm sorry.'

'What for?'

'I don't know.' And from across the room I looked at myself and shook my head in disbelief.

With love there comes an electricity between two people. Sometimes it sparks and brings passion – always it provides warmth. When it seems that it is switched off it brings an awkwardness and a formality that is hell, especially when one has to sit the other down on a lavatory seat.

Then one night we watched television in bed. Jim Rockford was in all kinds of trouble. The girl came from a rich family, spoilt rotten she was, and Jim's dad had warned him against her – but you know what Jim's like. He hadn't, however, reckoned on the Mafia connection, and neither had we, and we decided to leave the second half until the morning.

We settled down with a polite kiss and, with our backs to each other, pretended to sleep. Eventually sleep came, and then shots rang out and a car screamed across the dressing table on two wheels. I was out of bed in an instant, crouching by the wardrobe and searching for my gun in my shoulder holster. It wasn't there – I was naked.

Jim was being frisked by a woman cop outside a deserted warehouse and across the street four mafiosi sat in a Cadillac, frustrated in their efforts to waste him. They turned their heads and saw me, naked by the wardrobe – they moved towards me and the sweat poured down my face.

And then Diana rolled over in bed and, finding

the remote control stuck under her bottom, switched it off. She stared through the half-light and then, as the sleep fell away from her eyes, she saw me pressed against the wardrobe. At first she just shook – the bedclothes heaving with silent laughter – and then it roared to the surface. I fell upon her and we laughed and cried together – kissing and crying and laughing. And then we made love with a gentle passion and the electricity was earthed and for the first time in over a week I wasn't standing across the room watching me.

Sally came home early for Christmas with exciting news. 'How do you fancy having a croupier for a daughter?'

Well, it was all right by me – here was another skill we could learn together. By the time Sally qualified as a beauty therapist, I was theoretically brilliant. My anatomy had come on in leaps and bounds – I knew every bone in the body and every muscle and its function. I could quite easily have dissected a human body, and probably put it back together again.

At second hand I had learned about cathiodermy, electrolysis and the various diseases that we beauty therapists would have to be on the look-out for in our future patients. I was particularly good on moisturizers and the waxing of bikini lines. The only difference between us was that she could do the job and I couldn't. I looked forward to becoming a croupier – we were to begin our training in a Birmingham casino after Christmas.

It was a time for celebration and I was dispatched to the cellar for a couple of bottles of wine. It's not really a cellar – it used to be a coal place and now we kept the tumble dryer and the wine rack in there. There were six bottles to choose from. One was a peppermint cordial that I had won in a raffle at Longford village fête four years earlier, and two others turned out to be vinegar – one of these had a small tree growing inside it, and I was about to throw it away until Sally informed me that it was supposed to be in there. The fourth bottle contained cooking oil, but the fifth and sixth were red wine that I had laid down over a fortnight ago – I like to keep a good selection.

I opened the first bottle – it was an amusing little number and it had cost £1.69 per sparkling litre.

I said to Diana, 'There's all cork in the top of this bottle.'

'I know,' she said. 'They put it there to stop the wine running out.'

'No, what I mean is – there are all little bits of cork floating in the neck of the bottle.'

'You always do that,' Sally butted in. 'Either that or you push it down to the bottom.'

'It was a plastic screw top,' I told her. 'How can it have little pieces of cork floating about in it?'

'You worry too much about these things,' said Diana. 'Just pour me a glass and stop fussing.'

I poured a glass and handed it to Diana – she sniffed to savour the bouquet and her eyes watered.

'There are all little bits of cork floating in this,' she complained, handing me back the glass.

'That's what I've been trying to tell you – do you think I should take it back?'

'Strain it through a pair of my tights,' suggested Sally. 'That's what we do.' She seemed to have picked up some rather common habits down in London. 'Mind you, it's better if it's white wine – then you can wear the tights again afterwards.'

'I'm not drinking anything that's been strained through your tights,' declared Diana. 'Haven't we anything else? What about that bottle your mother gave us?'

'She hasn't given us any wine.'

'On your birthday – she brought you a parcel shaped like a bottle.'

'That was a thing for holding a lavatory brush.'

'Oh, yes – whatever happened to that? I haven't seen it since your mother left.'

'She took it back with her. She asked if we had a brush that would fit it, and when I said we hadn't she said that she had and she took it back with her.'

'Then why did she bring it in the first place?'

'You told her she shouldn't have,' Sally butted in.

'Well, she hasn't now, has she? She's taken it back. Now what about this wine?'

Sally had a theory about the cork. 'Maybe it came

over in one of those big tanker lorries, and to keep it from splashing all over the road they bung a cork in the tank.'

'I don't think so,' I said. 'It sounds a bit basic.'

'If you two don't mind,' said Diana, 'I would like a glass of wine.'

'I'll see to it,' said Sally.

'Not through your tights,' I warned her.

'No – the cork's floating on the top. I shall pour it from the bottom.' I followed her into the kitchen – I wanted to see this.

She poured the wine into a large jug and then through a sieve into another. It was looking better now, but still a flotilla of tiny cork lifeboats bobbed about on the surface.

She grabbed a leaf of kitchen roll and blotted the wine, but still the surface was littered with debris and so she dived into her handbag and, producing a pair of tights, proceeded to strain the wine back into the bottle.

'*Voilà*!' she cried as she filled a glass with wine as clear as a bell, and then she rinsed her tights under the tap and hung them over a radiator – the red stain standing out like the flag over the Kremlin.

'As long as I don't bend over, nobody will see that,' she declared triumphantly.

'Well, I don't fancy it now,' I grumbled as she marched off with a glass for her mother.

'We poured the other bottle away,' she told Diana, 'and opened a fresh one.' She never used to tell lies like that when she was little – but then she didn't wear tights when she was little either.

Diana took a sip and we waited eagerly. 'What's it taste like?'

'I've never tried Domestos,' she answered, 'but I imagine that it would have a similarly nectareous quality – it sort of thumps when it hits your stomach.'

'Let me have a sip,' begged Sally.

'Get your own,' said Diana, taking another sip and wincing.

A couple of hours later we settled down to the late-night movie.

'Any more wine?' Diana wanted to know.

'I'll get it,' offered Sally.

'You sit down – I'll do it,' I told her. After watching her previous performance I didn't trust her as far as I could throw her.

I opened a far more expensive bottle this time – I'd paid almost two pounds for this one and I wanted it done right. I unscrewed the plastic top and lined up three glasses, and into the first poured just a smidgin for a taste. It was a red wine – or at least I think it was. It was difficult to see it through the cork floating on the top.

I put my head round the door. 'Sally,' I whispered, and like a well-trained labrador she came bounding towards me.

'Yes?'

'Do me a favour, love – pass me the sieve and the two pyrex jugs, and do you think I could borrow your tights?'

Diana spent the run-up to Christmas in bed with Mavis Nicholson and friends, whilst Sally organized the coming feast and Nick and I tied up various bits of business and scoured Derbyshire and South Yorkshire for pickled walnuts.

Diana prepared lists, and Sally translated them into real terms.

'Right – who's going near a big Marks & Spencer's?'

'That's me.'

'There you are, then, Nick – leave the creams until Christmas Eve. Dad!'

'Yes?'

'You've got the bits and pieces, and don't forget to pick up Nana from the station.'

It had been the first night away from home in seven years for my mother – a funeral in London. She hadn't wanted to go.

'I can't leave the cat.'

'I can look after Whisky.'

'He'll need feeding.'

'I can open a tin of Whiskas.'

'Yes, but you don't know how much sugar he likes on it.'

*

The train pulled in on time and I watched as my mother stepped out of the end carriage and walked towards the shunting yards. I caught up with her and turned her round.

'How did it go?'

'All right – I didn't sleep very well. They had one of those duvet things.'

'You didn't like it?'

'I had to undo ten buttons before I could get inside it – in the end I just lay with it on top of me. It was just as effective.'

The buying of presents was a highly organized under-cover operation. With just a few days to go it became clear that Diana was not going to make it to the shops, and the kids and I were each sent out on a secret mission. I was to buy Sally's present from Diana, Nick was to buy mine and Sally was to buy Nick's. We set out together and then split like the Red Arrows – the first to finish was to join the queue outside Thornton's Chocolate Kabin.

I finished first and sat drinking coffee at a restaurant table – from there I could see the Thornton's queue backing up to the High Street. I watched as Nick bolted himself on to the tail – I would let the youngest handle the chocolates and join them later. Sally arrived to stand with him and, pleased that he now had company, I turned back to *Private Eye* and ordered another coffee.

To my list of presents I had added a special gift for Diana – a tin of Dulux white gloss. In January I had emulsioned the staircase and hall, but the paintwork was still a four-year-old white-gone-yellow – she would be thrilled.

'What! Two days before Christmas?' She wasn't as thrilled as I thought she'd be.

'I can finish it in the day – might as well do it while Sally's here.'

I am not a dab hand with doors. I paint them over and over again until, like the monkey with the typewriter, I seem to have achieved a finish without runs. By night-time I had completed four doors – each one a gleaming white complete with creases. The skirting board, however, remained untouched. I might perhaps have finished it had it not been for the kitchen shelf. Sally found the kit tucked away underneath her bed.

'Why not put this up? Mum would be chuffed – only take a couple of minutes.'

It took an hour and a half, but it did look well. Sally was almost pleased with the result.

'It's not quite level – but it'll do.'

'What do you mean it's not level?'

'It tilts to the right.'

'It's absolutely spot on.'

To prove my point I placed a tennis ball on the shelf, and it immediately rolled off the end.

'Never mind,' Sally comforted me. 'The cups won't roll off the end.' And they didn't – not unil she switched on the washing machine, whereupon they hurled themselves off the end like lemmings.

On Christmas Eve morning I made an early assault on the skirting board, and by ten the landing and stairs were finished – just the hall to go.

'Don't forget the fruit and vegetables,' shouted Diana. 'It's all gone by lunchtime today.'

I cleaned the paint from my hands and hair and teeth, changed my shoes and I was ready.

'Right, I'm off.'

She was working at her embroidery and the going was hard. The abstract picture was slowly coming to life with its rich red and golden kid, the gold wire stitches and the hundreds of tiny beads tumbling across velvet.

'This is a difficult bit.'

Her fingers were not strong enough to force the needle through the kid – she would place it in position and I would push it through, then pull it from the back. Then, after she had selected her spot, I would force the needle back to her. We worked together for a while, she the craftsman, me the labourer, until she could move on to an easier section.

'The vegetables.'

'Yes – I'm off.'

Watching her work on her embroidery always seemed to highlight the cruelty of this malevolent disability. She had so much talent in so many ways, and now this crippling virus was draining it all away from her.

We had kept only her early work. As her talent had matured she had sold her pictures. This one we would keep – it could be the last.

'The vegetables.'

'All right – you'll stay in bed, won't you?'

'Of course.'

'I shan't be long.'

Outside Statham's the greengrocers in Crown Square I took a deep breath and prepared myself. There was a pattern to my visits – a ritual. First I would be insulted by Beryl Statham, who owned the shop with husband George.

'Well, look who it is – star of stage, screen and radio. Heard you on Friday – what a load of old rubbish.'

I loved Beryl dearly and I always took her on and I always came second – a bad second. If I ever looked like winning, then her right-hand man Billy Clay would take me apart. He had a moustache that made Jimmy Edwards look like Ronald Colman and a voice that rattled the Matlock Hills. For years he had dominated the open market across the road, and now he had come in out of the cold.

They did their usual demolition job on me, and then I was allowed into the inner sanctum where George, sitting on a stool, was plucking geese. The stool was hidden by his immense bulk so that he seemed to be sitting in mid-air, and the geese looked like sparrows in his enormous hands.

George told me stories – fact and fiction. Horror stories from the Council chambers and delightful tales of Matlock past. Today it was the saga of the Ible chicken races and I left the shop, spitting feathers, with Friday's broadcast already written.

I had stayed too long. As I pushed open the door and laid the cardboard box on the draining board I heard Diana from the hallway.

'Don't worry – I'm all right.'

I ran from the kitchen and saw her lying on the floor. She had half draped the dustsheet around her like a sari, and crawled away from the stairs towards the kitchen door.

'I only fell halfway.'

I knelt beside her – no bruises on her face this time. Perhaps she had got away with it.

'I think I've broken my arm.'

I gently unwound the sari. Her left forearm was sticking out at an amazing angle – like a stick seen through water.

'Come on – let's get you to the hospital.'

'Sod it – I've got paint on my dressing gown.'

I lifted her to her feet and then picked her up in my arms. Her eyes were wandering now and she laid her head on my shoulders.

'Why?' I asked.

'I just wanted to be downstairs on my own – with nobody keeping an eye on me.'

I moved towards the door, taking care not to brush the broken arm against the frame.

'You haven't noticed, have you?'

'Noticed what?'

'While I was lying there I finished off the skirting board for you – I could only do so far up the door frame, I couldn't reach. But it's a help, isn't it?'

At the Chesterfield Royal we saw our usual doctor – the one who always dealt with our bruises and breaks.

'What happened this time?'

'He hit me again.'

The student nurse gave me a look full of loathing and disgust.

'Just 'cos his jelly wasn't set.'

They kept her in. She didn't object – she seemed to have forgotten that tomorrow was Christmas morning, and after her arm was set and plastered she was only too grateful to be tucked up between the crisp white sheets. I rang the kids and they came hurrying down, but she was already asleep when they arrived and after a while we left.

At my mother's we held a conference. Christmas would be postponed until further notice. The turkey would be held over and the brussels left uncooked – my mother's annual bottle of Asti

Spumante would remain unopened until Diana could share it with us.

This we pledged – with one exception. Whisky would be allowed his tin of salmon. My mother had argued his case eloquently – he wouldn't understand, she said. She had waved it under his nose every morning for a fortnight and he was now so excited she was afraid he might burst.

At home the kids had already tidied up the hall. The dustsheet was folded, the steps stacked away and the paintbrushes cleaned. But I brought them out again and finished off the door frame. When I stood back to examine the result there was a definite line roughly eighteen inches above the floor, where my new paint met Diana's old. To have produced a seamless finish I should have had to cover her handiwork, and I couldn't bring myself to do that.

It was the sort of line that might have measured the progress of a growing child – but it measured something entirely different, something not quite so tangible.

We breakfasted on Farley's rusks and cornflakes. I had suggested eggs and bacon, but Nick pointed out that the bacon was of the streaky variety and should by rights have been draped over the turkey. It was immediately disqualified by a majority vote of two to one.

With an eye to future meals I searched the pantry,

and after shuffling through the massed packets and jars of pickles, redcurrant jelly and chestnut stuffing I came to the conclusion that eggs would form the greater part of our diet over the next day or so – along with tinned tomatoes and beans.

It was a long morning. The pile of presents clustered under the Christmas tree smiled up at us and wagged their tails, but we ignored them stead-fastly and eventually they settled down and dropped off to sleep again.

As we parked outside the hospital we mingled with the lunchtime visitors. They were loaded down with gaily wrapped parcels and we felt quite inade-quate with just the spare nightie, the make-up bag and the quarter of Thornton's rum truffles. Perhaps we had misjudged the situation – but then if they let us take her home, all would be well.

As we climbed the first flight of stairs we were accompanied by a gorilla. He was pleasant enough – for a gorilla – and then on the first landing we were joined by a McDonald's clown and a beefburger. The three of them chatted amicably until we reached the door of Diana's ward, and then the gorilla's bleeper went off.

'Damn it,' he cried, 'I was going to chat up the bird in the black nightie,' and then he disappeared down the corridor. For a moment we considered the fate of a heart patient about to be given the kiss of life by a gorilla.

Then the McDonald's clown held the door open for the beefburger and I followed through – anxious to chat up the bird in the black nightie.

She was sitting up in bed, a radiant smile on her face. She wore a paper hat of many colours and in her right hand was a glass of red wine. On a tray in front of her was a Christmas dinner with all the trimmings, and a Christmas pudding waited in the wings.

Sally looked at Nick – I looked at Sally – and Nick looked at the both of us. We were thinking of the eggs and beans and tomatoes. We moved a tangle of streamers from the bed and sat on the edge. Diana gave me a lovely smile and while I kissed her Sally stole a small sausage from her plate.

Her dinner looked quite appetizing for hospital fare. There was something I didn't quite recognize lurking by the sprouts – it looked as though it had just crawled out of the ocean and was contemplating life on earth, but the turkey lay tender and tempting.

'Better eat your dinner, love,' and I began to cut it into bite-sized pieces, 'then I'll see if we can take you home.'

She smiled at Sally and said through a mouthful of turkey, 'I asked them, but they said not yet.'

I was sure I could persuade them that she would be well cared for at home – after all these years I was almost state registered.

'The turkey looks nice,' I said as she speared a chunky cube of white breast.

The fork paused in mid-air. 'Turkey?' she

exclaimed as she examined it at close quarters. 'I thought it was fish.'

On second thoughts, perhaps it might be best if she stayed in for another day or so – then we could begin all over again.

14

My mother put the first-aid box back on the shelf and pulled out the knife drawer.

'They'll not be in there – I keep them in here.' In my innocence I had thought that a first-aid box was the natural place to keep an aspirin, but I was wrong.

'That's for plasters and things – you don't keep aspirins in there.' She laid out first the forks on the draining board and then the spoons. 'They're in here somewhere.' The knives followed, and then the larger spoons and ladles until the drawer was empty. She was puzzled. 'I could have sworn they were in here.' And then a great beam came over her face.

'How silly of me – I had a clear out,' and with a confident air she opened the butter compartment in the fridge door and produced a single soluble aspirin.

'There you are. I've only got the one – if you're going to get all these headaches I'd better get some more.'

The headaches had been coming thick and fast lately – real belting headaches, revolving eyeballs and the lot.

'You're not getting enough sleep, that's what it is.' She was tearing at the foil wrapping and getting nowhere. 'And you don't eat enough to keep a sparrow alive.'

Suddenly the soluble aspirin flirted out of the foil, shot six inches in the air, landed on her foot and bounced under the fridge. I fell on my knees to retrieve it and found myself staring at a bread knife. She had obviously done this before and so I let her get on with it. She poked the knife under the fridge and with a great sweeping movement brought out about a pound and a half of fluff. Sifting carefully through it she found a button and a ping-pong ball before she recovered the aspirin and then, as I helped her to her feet, she examined it carefully.

'You can't swallow that – it's mucky,' and she moved over to the sink and washed my soluble aspirin under the tap.

We watched as it dissolved into a paste and disappeared down the plughole. After a moment's silence she wiped her hands on her apron and said, 'What you need is something to eat – do you a lot more good than aspirins.'

I shuffled the cutlery back in the drawer while she set about cooking me a *square* meal. That's what I needed, she said, 'A square meal.'

I suppose a boil-in-the-bag cod in butter sauce has got to be a square meal in every sense of the word, and she set about the preparation of this

211

delicacy with a confidence that stemmed from cooking little else over the past four years.

I watched in admiration as she first brought a pan of water to the boil and then gently slipped the bag beneath the angry waves.

'Not take long,' she said as she produced another bag from the fridge. 'You'll enjoy this – make a nice change.'

She slipped the second bag in alongside the first and chased them round with a wooden spoon.

'What are we having with it?' I asked, already knowing the answer.

'How do you mean?'

She didn't understand the question. For as long as I could remember we had taken our main course neat.

'Would you like a nice pork chop?' she would ask as I trotted in from school, and that's what I would have, a nice pork chop – nothing else, no vegetables, no chips.

'Keep an eye on that pan,' she ordered, handing me the spoon. 'Keep the bags moving – it's important.'

She disappeared, and returned almost immediately with a sprig of mint in her hand. She took charge of the spoon once more and then, with a Gallic flourish, dropped the mint into the boiling water.

'There,' she said, 'it makes all the difference.'

We sat at the long oak table that my father had made – she at one end, me at the other. The best knives and forks were laid out on the white damask tablecloth, and squatting on the Sunday plates were two small squares of fish.

'Have you any salt?'

'I've something very similar.' She went over to the sideboard and produced a small yellow drum.

'What is it?'

'Pepper.'

I pointed the car towards Matlock and she waved me off as though I were going to war. I had a hundred and fifty boxes of waist slips in the car – a dozen slips in each, and all for Henry Margolis in Manchester.

Henry would pay me on delivery, and I would be able to pay the wages tomorrow. Then I would buy more fabric, lace, elastic, thread, polythene bags and boxes so that I could make more slips for the Passmores or the Hiltons or the Nichols or maybe Henry again.

It was a merry-go-round that had long since stopped making money. I wasn't producing enough to make money – just enough to pay the wages and buy fabric and lace and boxes.

I needed to see if Diana was all right before I carried on to Manchester – I had arranged for a friend to look after her, but there was no car outside the house when I drew up.

'You go – I'll be all right.'

'I'll wait until she arrives – I've got plenty of time.'

213

It would take me about an hour and a half to drive over to Henry's – a little longer if I hit the rush hour.

'I'll stay in bed, I promise.'

She had been a little better these past few days – a month of solid rest had brought with it mixed results. She was stronger and had more energy, but the blackouts were coming thick and fast now and, as she grew more adventurous, so the danger increased.

'Honest – I'll stay in bed.'

I looked at my watch. 'I've still got half an hour before I need to go – I'll make us a drink.'

We sat and talked around many things without really talking about anything. I needed to be off now and I fought the temptation to keep glancing at my watch – I moved over to the other side of the bed from where I could see the clock on the video.

'It's time you were off.'

'I'm all right for a bit.'

The conversation was stilted, and it was my fault. For weeks now that feeling had crept back – that feeling of not being myself, of watching myself from across the room as someone else performed inside my shell.

My face seemed like a mask and I couldn't feel my cheekbones. That morning I had dug my fingernails into my face and felt nothing, and yet when I looked in the mirror there were the marks. When I smiled I had to work at it – to pull strings inside my head before my teeth would show.

I had met Paul Wolfenden earlier in the week. Paul and I had been a double act, he the comic, me the feed, and we had triumphed together and, even more often, died together on the stage. We were like brothers, and yet that day we were like a ventriloquist and his dummy and our delighted greetings had fallen away as I merely went through the motions.

Diana knew something was wrong, she didn't know what – but she was sure that it was her fault.

'Please go now – you'll miss Henry. You can be back in four hours – I'll be perfectly all right.'

'Promise to stay where you are.' I had to go or I couldn't pay the wages in the morning.

'Promise – just fill me a bottle, my feet are cold.'

I waited in the kitchen for the kettle to boil – I could just about make it. The rush-hour traffic would be thickening as I hit Manchester, but I had ten minutes to spare if all went well.

As I poured the water into the bottle there was a crash on the ceiling. I ran up the stairs and into the room.

She was lying unconscious, half in bed and half out. The bedside table was on its side – the table lamp rolled on the floor soaked in orange juice, and the phone buzzed into the carpet.

I pulled her back into bed and stroked each side of her neck until she came round. She blinked up at me – bewildered.

'I only reached for my drink.'

'You're all right now, love.'

She wasn't even safe in bed – I couldn't leave her. I made her comfortable and tidied up the mess. I'd have to ask the bank for the wages and suffer that look I was getting more and more as I offered what they obviously thought was yet another sob story.

'How much will you need?'

'Five hundred – I shall have a cheque in for almost two thousand on Monday.'

'Oh, that should bring the overdraft down a little.'

'No – not exactly. I have to buy fabric on Tuesday.'

'How much will you need for that?'

'Fifteen hundred.'

A pause. 'Perhaps we could see the accounts. . . .'

No, they couldn't – not yet. I'd seen a draft myself and I was not impressed. It was not the right time to try the bank – but how?

'Hullo – anybody home?' The cavalry arrived in the shape of Yvonne, a brand-new next door neighbour. I had talked to her over the fence a couple of times – she had a husband, a young daughter and two stuck-up cats who each wore a collar and a supercilious expression.

'Yvonne – could you stay with me? Deric has to go.'

'Yes.' No hesitation – no having to think about it. I began to explain just why I needed to. . . .

'Go on – shove off.' She took the dishcloth from

my hand and began to tidy the things I had already tidied.

So I shoved off.

A stuffed parrot sat in the rear window of the caravan and leered at me as I tried to pass. The caravan lurched along the Via Gellia and swung its bum out across the narrow Roman road every time I tried my famous Emerson Fittipaldi manoeuvre. Further down the road some tortured soul was dispatching cars at regular intervals so that they clogged up the straight bits, and eventually I admitted defeat and tried to ignore the gloating parrot.

I often wrote my radio pieces in the car. An hour and a half behind the wheel would produce a rough five minutes to be polished later on the typewriter.

This was my last chance to draft something for the 'Line Up' programme tomorrow. What was it Ashley wanted? 'It's National Sock Week, Deric – thought it was right up your street.'

What the hell could I do with National Sock Week? I could do something on Strangle-a-Parrot-Week. Think – come on, think. Bloody caravans, I'll never get there on time. National Sock Week – hope Diana's all right, I didn't take her to the toilet before I left – why didn't she say something? When I get past this caravan I'll slew the car right across its path, force it off the road and beat that parrot to death. Forty-seven minutes – I'll never make it in forty-seven minutes. What's the bank manager's name? Come on, you bastard – pull over!

The parrot turned left and I turned right towards Buxton – OK, let's go! Thirty-nine minutes – I shan't make it now. How can I pay the wages? Can't be funny for tomorrow – everything is falling apart – not enough time to do anything properly. 'You could always sell the house,' the bank manager had said – Diana would hate that. Think about National Sock Week. God! my head hurts – it's bursting and my face is stiff – I can't feel it. . . . I was watching myself again.

The man pulled the car over on to the verge and switched off the engine. He sat for a while, his head in his hands, and then he opened the door and climbed out. I watched him as he clambered over the wall and began to walk across the fields which soon gave way to rough moorland.

He didn't see the ditch – he just walked straight through it, up to his knees in muddy water. He said that his head hurt – there was so much in there whirling around and around. Did I know that National Sock Week started tomorrow and that it was very, very funny? He'd never get to Henry now. He didn't want to sell his house, Diana loved it, but he would have to – he couldn't think straight, you see, thoughts tumbled over one another and crashed into one another and he couldn't sort them out. He had the accounts to do and the windows hadn't been cleaned for weeks and cups rolled off the end of the shelf – did I know it was National Sock Week and that his wife was ill? She had some tablets in a boot polish tin. He hadn't found the others.

It was getting dark now and he must have walked for an hour or more, stumbling here and there as he tired and then he tried to climb another wall. A country road ran alongside the wall and he seemed surprised to see it. As he climbed his foot caught on the topmost stones and he fell, landing on his knees on the far side.

For a few moments he didn't move – knees on the grass, hands on the tarmac fringe. And then he began to cry, tears running down his face, and the crying turned to sobbing and it seemed that he would never stop. He was pathetic.

I couldn't stop crying. I hadn't cried for ages – I gulped now and then at happy endings, and I'd fought back the tears many times as Diana fought her battles. Once we had cried together, arms folded around each other, as we had tried to talk calmly about the future.

But nothing like this. I sobbed uncontrollably and it frightened me – the sobs came right up from my shoes. My shoes – what had happened to my shoes? They were soaking – it went right up to my knees. God, I was a mess.

Across the road a white Cortina slowed down and stopped and a man got out. He was a big man. He wore blue mechanic's overalls and he was watching me. I couldn't get up and I lowered my head and stared down at the grass.

I heard his feet crunch as he walked towards me –
I saw his knees as he squatted and then his hand as he
placed it on my arm. It was tattooed, a blue and red
eagle – he wouldn't understand a man crying.

'Come on,' he lifted me to my feet and walked me
over to the car. 'Get in.'

'I'm dirty.'

'Get in.'

We sat for some time in silence. He switched the
heater on and I wiped my face with my hands – at
least I'd stopped crying.

'Do you want a doctor?'

'No – I must get home.'

'Where's that?'

'Matlock.'

'How did you get here?'

'A car.' I had no idea where I was, and when he
told me I was none the wiser. 'I was going towards
Buxton on the Ashbourne road – I walked from
over there.'

He drove down narrow lanes until we hit the
main road, and then he turned left towards Buxton.
After a few miles he turned round and we scoured
the road towards Ashbourne. The car was pulled
over on to the grass verge – the door hung wide
open, a hundred and fifty dozen waist slips getting
the benefit of the cold night air.

'Will you be all right?'

'Yes, thank you – thanks for everything.'

'I'll be off, then.' He waited until I started the car,

and then he swung round and disappeared towards Buxton. I spun the wheel and set off in the opposite direction.

I drove slowly – I was exhausted, mentally more than physically – what a pillock! Automatically I checked the rear view mirror and caught a glimpse of my face – it was filthy, streaked with mud where I'd wiped the tears away with my hands.

I also caught a glimpse of a white Cortina following at a respectful distance. I slowed down – the Cortina slowed. He followed me until I turned off the main road and back down the Via Gellia. I parked up and waited for him – he saw me and I stuck my arm out through the window in salute – he hit his horn and then swung the car round once again and disappeared.

I still felt very strange – nothing like this had ever happened to me before. My face was foam rubber and my eyes were tired, but my brain was now cold as ice. For the first time in months the fuzzy edges had gone and I could think clearly. Tomorrow I would nip over to the Passmores before breakfast – they would buy enough to pay the wages and I would sell this damn business. Sod the bank – I could earn a living as a writer. I was good enough, and if I wasn't I'd soon find out. I would start right now with five minutes on National Sock Week for the BBC. Be positive – think positive.

I turned the key in the ignition and the car wouldn't start.

15

Diana lay by the side of me, her breasts rising and falling with each breath – it was a sight I could watch for hours and a lovely way to start a new day. She shivered slightly and, with her elbow, pulled the sheet up almost to her neck. As her arm fell away I unwrapped her again and lay back and thought of England.

It had been a good week. Marjorie and Brian Passmore had received me gracefully over breakfast last Friday, and not batted an eyelid as I appeared from nowhere bearing one hundred and fifty dozen waist-slips.

The Passmores had built up their business from a single market stall, and they now had a turnover that would have many a department store wondering where they were going wrong. The two sons, Shaun and David, had joined the business and it was about to burst at the seams.

'If you ever think of selling the factory, Deric . . .'

'Now it's funny you should mention that.'

A month's rest seemed to have pumped energy into Diana and we had made sure that it wasn't wasted.

She had practised walking with her elbow crutches, and as long as I propped up her left leg we made steady, if painful, progress.

The sun had gone on overtime, and for long spells a sun-lounger replaced her bed and a clear blue sky her bedroom ceiling.

Sally had returned briefly from the casino school in Birmingham as a fully fledged croupier – a two-game dealer now she was, ready to be launched any day upon an innocent Manchester. She spent her time with us practising snoozing and dozing between bouts of fierce scrubbing, as she attempted to remove the dreaded basement green mould from her Tupperware containers in time for the move.

Nick and I had spent the previous evening playing cricket over in Etwall for the Radio Derby All Stars, and we had both made our mark. Nick had scored a match-winning fifty-six runs, and I had pulled a muscle. I was quite proud of the pulled muscle – in my thigh it was, and although it hurt like mad it was nice to know that there were still muscles there to be pulled.

John Kettley, the weatherman, had been about to bowl and I crouched behind the wicket, my trusty gloves at the ready – then Graham Wren, at first slip, had tapped me on the shoulder and attempted to sell me a raffle ticket. That sort of thing does nothing for the concentration, and as the ball whistled past my ear I flung myself violently to the ground and pulled a muscle.

I would work on a more noble version of the incident for Diana's benefit, but in the meantime, thanks to Nick's half-century, we had won by a couple of runs.

I limped off the pitch with John Kettley.

'Close, wasn't it?'

'Yes,' he agreed, 'very warm.'

We had travelled home in Nick's car, as the *Derbyshire Times* paid for his petrol whilst I had to pay for my own. I wanted to talk about my muscle, but Nick was full of his half-century.

'I think the shot that gave me the most pleasure was that straight drive for four.'

'I didn't see that – but then I was probably off having treatment.'

'I knew it was a four, the moment it left my bat.'

I gave up and, apart from the odd theatrical wince, let him work through his triumph stroke by stroke. Eventually he ran out of runs and changed the subject.

'Jo and I are thinking of getting married in September – how do you feel about it?'

I had been waiting for this ever since they had become engaged a few months ago and assured us that they would wait at least another couple of years.

'It's fine by me – but don't you think you're a bit young?'

'We're older than you and Mum were when you got married.'

I had been waiting for that one as well – I hate it when people fight dirty.

'That was different. I was in the forces - I might never have come back.'

'You were doing your National Service in Hereford.'

'Yes - well. What does Jo think her mum and dad will say?'

'They're quite happy – we asked them last night.'

'Oh! Well, as I say, it's fine by me. Just let me have a word with your mum first.'

'She's all in favour.'

'When did you tell her?'

'While you were getting changed to come out – she said she'd have a word with you first.'

'Right – well, congratulations. September, you said?'

'Yes.' He hesitated, wondering how to put it. 'I didn't want to leave it too long – just in case anything happened to Mum. I want her to be there.'

We were quiet for a moment or so as we pulled up outside the house.

'I think it's a good idea. You have my blessing, my son – and Nick . . .'

'Yes?'

'Thank you for asking my permission.'

It was summer dark as we had walked down the

drive, and my Citroën lay sprawled under the carport. As we drew closer I noticed a sheet of white paper sellotaped to the windscreen. I couldn't have got a ticket – not in my own drive.

It was a page torn from a notebook and I took it in the kitchen and switched on the light.

'*The leg on the front of the wheelbarrow is wonky.*'

I didn't have a wheelbarrow. I read it again and then passed it to Nick.

'Maybe it's in code,' he suggested, 'like in "Secret Army". They say "The leg on the front of the wheelbarrow is wonky", and you have to answer, "The tattoo on your left buttock is that of a small porcupine."'

I didn't think it likely. The only underground movement we had in Matlock were the potholers – and I was too tired to think, anyway, and my pulled muscle was playing me up.

'I'm off to bed – I'll work it out in the morning.' I paused in the hallway. 'Nick – I'm glad about the wedding . . .'

'Thanks, Dad.' He sounded genuinely pleased.

' . . . and congratulations on the fifty – I was proud of you.'

'Thanks.'

I paused on the first step, my pulled muscle whimpering, waiting for a simple word of sympathy.

'I'll be up myself in a minute, Dad – just have a Weetabix.'

And I hope it chokes you, I thought, as I hobbled up the stairs.

And so this morning, as I lay beside Diana and contemplated her breasts, I felt very happy and contented. She had been much better this last month – still the hands had to be clamped in wire and plaster and still the pain was there, but keeping her free from exhaustion by excluding even the smallest task had paid a dividend. The exhaustion dampened her mind and intensified the pain. With the rest, her brain had sharpened and she wasn't searching for words as she had before – the saving grace had been the sun.

Apart from a cross-bedroom session with the elbow-crutches each morning she was doing absolutely nothing – no embroidery, no painting of nails – and this idleness would have had her at screaming point had it not been for the sunshine.

Even years ago, when she had the constitution of a small horse, she would lie in the sun for hours on end, only turning now and then to facilitate an even tan. Had we been able to roast her on a spit, her happiness would have been complete. So now she soaked up the sunshine and the world was good. The warmth comforted her icy feet and hands and charged her body with well-being. The problems would come when the weather changed – but for the time being everything in the garden was lovely, especially Diana.

*

I leaned across and stroked the nearest breast — nothing too strenuous, my pulled muscle was waking up and demanding attention.

I hadn't told her about my walk across the moors, but she guessed that something had happened — I had come home rather shell-shocked and, although I'd managed to wash and change, I hadn't been able completely to wipe the stunned expression from my face.

I felt at peace once more — the tension had eased and the mask had fallen away. He still watched me now and then, but not with such a critical eye, and I was able to be myself again.

Diana was awake and turning towards me, 'Morning – how was the cricket?'

'We won.'

'Good God!'

'Nick scored a half-century.'

'What about you?'

'I pulled a muscle,' I rubbed my thigh. 'It's very stiff.'

'That's how I like it.' She rolled over towards me.

I slid out of bed and hobbled over to the door. 'I can't stand crude women.'

'It's your turn to make the coffee.'

It had been my turn to make the coffee every morning for the past twenty-six years. I pulled on a pair of trousers and limped downstairs. As the kettle boiled I sat at the table and read the paper back to front, leaving the politics until I felt stronger. Something wasn't quite right – a movement through the French windows caught my eye and I turned to look.

I couldn't believe it. The patio, if that's the correct term for seven paving stones, was covered in flowers. There were one, two, three – seven tubs packed with exotic blooms, and three hanging baskets quivered from the carport. It looked like Kew Gardens – it was an incredible sight. The one sure thing was that they weren't ours – we had a hanging basket back and front. This new display was a veritable Burmese jungle, and I wouldn't have been at all surprised if a Japanese soldier had emerged from the foliage and given himself up.

I opened the French windows and stepped out into Fantasy Island. Apart from the tubs and baskets there was a small trough full of miniature roses and an ornamental dwarf wheelbarrow packed to the brim with fuchsias.

'What a stupid place to put a wheelbarrow,' I thought. 'Somebody could trip over that,' and I took hold of the handles and pushed it a yard nearer the fence. I let go of the handles and it fell over.

I remembered the note on my windscreen: '*The leg on the front of the wheelbarrow is wonky.*' Well, it wasn't wonky now – it had fallen off. I jammed it back under the barrow and went upstairs.

'Have you seen our patio?' I asked Diana.

'Do your zip up,' she ordered.

'What are all these flowers?'

'They're from Rosie and Keith.'

I was overcome. They had sent Diana a bunch of chrysanthemums when she fell downstairs at Christmas, but this was unbelievable. How could they possibly have heard about my pulled muscle? Never mind, it was a gesture I should never forget – perhaps Keith had experienced a pulled muscle himself and knew how painful it was.

'They've brought them round for you to water while they are on holiday,' said Diana, and another crumb of comfort was hoovered away.

'Wouldn't it have been easier for me to go round there?' I asked her. 'It would have saved the plants the trauma of a journey into the unknown and probably saved Keith from a hernia.'

'It's the police,' said Diana.

Good God, I thought, they must have fallen off the back of a lorry – we could be done for receiving.

'The police told Rosie and Keith that there are thieves going around stealing hanging baskets and whatever – then they sell them at car boot sales for ten pounds a time.'

At that rate we had some two hundred and fifty pounds' worth of prize blooms sunning themselves on our patio. Tonight I would have to ride shotgun, and since the pollen count in the garden must now be standing at around seven thousand that wasn't going to be easy – and me with a pulled muscle.

★

As we drove through Rowsley towards Bakewell we felt like a couple of kids out on the loose. It was as though I'd just passed my driving test and thrown away the L plates, and Diana had turned sixteen five minutes ago and they couldn't touch us for it any more. We felt a freedom we hadn't felt for years – there was no wheelchair in the boot. Just a couple of sticks on the back seat, and we'd tied ribbons round the handles to celebrate. Field Farm and the Moneys' party awaited us.

We had started out to so many parties and had to abort the mission halfway down the stairs – tonight Diana had dressed in a little black number, tarted up with too much gold jewellery.

'I can't decide between this – or this. What do you think?'

'Wear the lot.'

We had done the nails between us – just a touch of lipstick, and the golden tan meant that the blusher could stay sealed in its jar. It had been so easy, and she had shimmied down the stairs on her bottom without so much as a groan.

In the hall she had used me as a prop, my two hands on her bottom as she stood and surveyed herself in the mirror. I knelt down low on the floor so that there was no reflection of me – just a woman in a black dress with an arm sticking strangely out of her rear end. We shuffled forwards so that the flat shoes wouldn't ruin the picture – the six-inch high heels with the sexy thin straps were

231

already in the car, but they were only for sitting down in.

No matter how much you spend on that little black dress, it was designed to swing or cling as the case may be and not to have the life squeezed out of it in a wheelchair. She delighted in this reincarnation of her old self.

'Just another button, I think.'

I had sat her down on the stairs and undone another button. This had been her major weapon in the wheelchair. There are few advantages in living life at navel level and they have to be exploited for all they are worth.

At parties you are stuck in the chair and, like a moth to a flame, you attract the most boring man in the world who sits by you for ever and talks of his cycling holiday in the Lake District.

But a low-cut neckline at first-floor level can be devastating. Diana had long since thrown away her bra, and a couple of extra buttons craftily undone meant that she always had half a dozen men standing high above her, gazing down with eyeballs on full throttle.

'What a delightful necklace.'

'Can I get you another drink?'

But tonight a single button would suffice. She felt confident and happy – it was a heady experience and she wasn't used to it. Tonight she sat in the passenger seat and looked forward to an evening where a normal conversation wouldn't be a battle of will.

Fred's hands did nothing for the outfit, but she had clipped several pairs of earrings to the wire struts, and the diamante sparkled against the plaster I had polished specially for the occasion.

'Deric – do you think many people will turn up at my funeral?'

'I'm sure of it – I shall certainly make a point of being there myself.'

Even her conversation reminded me of the old days – the bizarre opening gambits that never failed to surprise me.

'I want Ian Gregory to conduct the service – I think he likes me – and for music I want Andy Fairweather-Lowe singing "Wide Eyed and Legless".'

'Seems very appropriate.'

That settled, she cast a critical eye over the little black dress and undid another button – just to be on the safe side.

There was a rumour – I didn't believe it for a moment – that an underground pipeline from Harrods ran all the way up the M1 and surfaced at Fields Farm just by that little rockery next to the swimming pool. Certainly most of the goodies I piled high on Diana's plate hadn't come out of a square box to be cooked at 180 degrees for twenty-five minutes, but then they didn't have a Marks & Spencer's in Bakewell.

'I'll have something of everything,' Diana had

ordered, and I plundered the fresh salmon, the Scotch beef and the roast pork and garnished it with pickles that were strange to my untrained eye. She would find it tame fare after my Cumberland Pie, I thought, as I carried the plates over to where she held court by the fireplace.

I put a plate in front of her on the coffee table and listened to the conversation as I concentrated on my own plate, cutting first my beef and then my pork into small square cubes. Diana picked up her knife carefully and then waved it in the air to illustrate a point.

I boned my salmon with a fork, opened it up a bit for easy access, and then cut the larger pickles until they were smaller pickles.

She picked up her fork and moved in on her plate – she paused.

'Is there any apple sauce?'

'Sorry.'

I disappeared for a moment with the plates and then returned, the fault corrected.

'There you are.'

'Thank you.' She smiled and then, laying down the knife, she aimed her fork and began to spear the tailor-made cubes.

Teamwork, that's what it was. We had perfected the switch over a number of years so that she wouldn't have to sit there, waiting like a two-year-old, whilst I cut up her meat.

★

We danced for the first time in years, or at least we stood there, tottering, while others danced around us and Nat King Cole rambled on about his rose.

I had never been able to dance – I did a slow waltz to everything. If the band played a quickstep, I heated up my slow waltz a couple of degrees and tried to keep up with the others, but it was no good.

I once took lessons in the quickstep and would appear quite proficient until somebody spoke to me – then my legs collapsed. I had to concentrate on the music to the exclusion of all else – one 'Do you come here often?' reduced my legs to a jelly, and I would mutter something about my war wound and retire to the bar.

I also had a habit of dancing backwards, allowing the woman to lead – it was something I didn't like to analyze too closely.

Diana had been a splendid dancer once, but now she had slumped down to my level and, as Neil Diamond moved on to centre stage and tried to up the tempo with the 'Reggae Strut', it seemed like a good time to call it a night.

At home we sat out amidst the pot-plant jungle and savoured the taste of old times. Diana had to be carried out of the car and the old familiar exhaustion was sweeping back over her, but she was reluctant to call an end to a day that had once more brought her back into the real world.

'I forgot to tell you – your mother rang.'

'Is she all right?'

'Yes – she just rang to say her phone was out of order.'

It was a new phone – a tacky-green slimline model, so light and plasticky after the black heavyweight she had housed for years that she held it between finger and thumb for fear it might break.

'How did she ring us if her phone's out of order?'

'Well – she says she can ring us, but she can't ring anyone else. Her line's gone stiff – but she rings us so often that the line between us must have eased.'

'That makes sense.'

'She wanted to know if I thought she was squeezing the phone too hard.'

'What did you say?'

'I asked if she was wearing rubber gloves.'

'And was she?'

'Yes – I told her to take them off and she said it was perfect then.'

'Probably the static.'

'That's what she thought.'

It was just like old times – the heady scent of flowers in bloom, the intoxicating aroma of hot chocolate and the cut and thrust of intelligent conversation.

'Did she say anything else?'

'Yes – she'd like you to pop round tomorrow. She says she's illegitimate and it's time that you were told.'

16

Diana needed my full attention on the Sunday. The party had taken its toll and she was totally exhausted. Hot baths and hot bottles helped to ease the pain, but the disturbed vision and the violent headaches were even more worrying, as was the difficulty she had with her words. She lay with a cold flannel over her eyes and tried to tell Sally how well she had done the night before.

'It was lovely, Sally. We . . . er . . . I . . . and your dad, we . . . er . . . .' A big effort now. 'The . . . heels, high heels and . . . it was . . . .' A sad shake of the head. 'Your dad – he'll . . . tell you.'

I told Sally as we sat on either side of the bed, and Sally listened and held Diana's hand.

It was early evening before I left her to drive into Chesterfield. A quick visit to the factory – the pressure had lifted there. I was teaching the Passmores the ropes and they were learning a lot faster than I had done. They would take over shortly, and then perhaps I would have time.

My mother was waiting for me in the garden – Whisky sat at her side, plastered from head to paw in grass cuttings.

237

'You'll never guess what I've done.'

'You've cut through the electric cable with the mower.'

'How did you know that?'

When she had first bought the mower from the Co-op, the electric cable had reached right down to the end of the garden, but she had sliced through it so often that it was now only about twelve feet long. The power point was just inside the garage and she could only mow as far as the birdbath. Today, however, she had surpassed herself – she had actually sliced through the cable whilst the mower was still in the garage. She watched me splice together what there was left to splice together.

'Wouldn't you think they'd put a longer lead on them?'

'If you remember – they did,' I told her as I hauled my extension cable out of the car. My mother eyed it lovingly – it was a beauty, a hundred and fifty yards on a winding reel, and I was very proud of it.

'It's handy you happened to have it with you, isn't it?' she said. 'If you left it here, I could use it.'

That's how I had lost the last one. She had whittled it down by the hour and I had discovered the last twenty yards, coiled under her bed, servicing her electric blanket.

I mowed the lawn and clipped the edges. I did this every week – maybe she wasn't as daft as I thought she was. She had a pot of tea waiting for me as I finished, and we sat looking at the garden.

'What do hedgehogs eat?' she asked as I swirled the sugar around in my cup.

'Slugs, I think – and worms.'

'Ugh – they can't enjoy it, can they?'

'There's no accounting for taste.'

We sat and watched Whisky as he washed himself and spat out blades of grass.

'Would a hedgehog eat bacon?'

'Depends on whether he was Jewish or not.'

'He doesn't look Jewish.' She sat up sharply and pointed to the lawn. 'There he is – look.' And sure enough, there in the half-light was a young hedgehog, sniffling across the grass.

'He's only a baby, isn't he?'

'I call him Eric. I've burnt some bacon – do you think he'd like it?'

'You'd be better off with bread and milk.'

She disappeared into the kitchen. 'Brown bread or white?'

'Brown – he looks as though he needs building up.'

The hedgehog was working the freshly clipped lawn edges, but at the sound of my mother quietly opening the French windows he was off like a shot.

'You're too late,' I told her as he scuttled off towards the bottom hedge. She hurled the windows wide open and yelled, 'Eric!' and the hedgehog stopped dead in his tracks.

I have often wanted to get a closer look at a hedgehog, with little success – but then I had never known one by its christian name before.

He hid under the hedge as she placed the bread and milk by the birdbath, and it must have been five minutes before he reappeared and made straight for the bowl. He tucked in as though he hadn't eaten for a week.

My mother looked puzzled. 'That's not Eric.'

'Of course it is.' I'd begun to think of him as Eric now.

'Eric isn't as grey as that – there!' She pointed to the far end of the lawn where three little hedgehogs were yomping their way through the hedge. 'That's Eric.'

Following immediately on their heels was a much larger hedgehog. 'That's Hilda - their mother.'

The whole gang were now circling the dish and the slurping was appalling. Five hedgehogs make more noise than you would hear in a Little Chef all week.

'I'm glad you told me about the bread and milk – they like it, don't they?'

Eric certainly did – he was swimming in the middle of the dish.

'Have you seen the father?'

'Geoff got run over last week,' she said, fighting back a tear as the one-parent family turned to go, leaving Eric to struggle out of the bowl on his own.

My mother lived in a wonderful world peopled by hedgehogs called Eric and lions who played with squirrels and in which big monkeys were told off for hitting small monkeys. But people were her favourite animals, and she would travel miles past her bus stop if she found herself seated alongside a promising specimen. Her chain of reasoning had the odd link missing, but this was what made her company so delightful.

'Mrs Morris can't be as blind as she makes out – she's taking her dog for a walk in the dark.'

No use pointing out that the dog was a guide dog and it was taking Mrs Morris for a walk and if she was blind it didn't matter that it was dark.

'Why do you always shout at Mrs Morris? She isn't deaf.'

'I know she isn't deaf – there wouldn't be any point in me shouting at her if she was deaf.'

Maybe there wasn't a link missing – maybe she had an extra link. Certainly every now and then she produced something that no one else had thought of.

'Do you remember Diana saying that she'd been very ill with polio as a girl and that it went on for a long time and they thought she was going to be paralyzed – and then it went, just like that? Well, I think that's got something to do with the way she is now.'

Who knows? Maybe my mother had something – maybe she hadn't. It wasn't a theory that I would care to put before the doctors. They would be sure to find holes in it – holes were all they had seemed to find so far.

'I know a lot of people who had that funny polio –
it wasn't the real thing and they've all suffered later in
life, one way and another.'

She pulled the curtains and shut out the night and
then came to sit closer to me.

'Anyway – there's something I want to tell you.
Do you remember your Auntie May?'

'Yes.'

'Well, she wasn't your Auntie May – she was your
grandma.'

'How do you mean?'

My mother had been one of seven sisters – May,
who had never married, was the eldest, my mother
the youngest.

'May got herself pregnant and it wasn't done in
those days – so they sent her away and when she came
back with me I was passed off as her baby sister. I'm
illegitimate.'

I felt very sad. May had been my baby-sitter and
had played with me for hours, but she was just one of
six aunties, no more than that – if I'd known she was
my grandmother I might have felt more for her.

'Does it make any difference?'

'No, of course not.'

'Good – only now that you're forty-eight I
thought you were old enough to know.'

I drove home wondering: 'Why forty-eight?' Did
one acquire an understanding that wouldn't have
been there at forty-seven? I had also discovered,

during her lurid description of May's seduction, that I was now one-quarter Jewish – I quite liked that. I had a two-shelf collection of books by Jewish writers and now I could read them as an insider – or, at least, one in every four.

I worried, though, about my extension cable. It was my pride and joy – a hundred and fifty yards long it was and on a winding reel and I had left it, alone and helpless, in my mother's garage. I wondered what length it would be by the time I picked it up.

For two and a half weeks Diana lay in a darkened room. It was a hell of a price to pay for a night out, but gradually she began to feel better and the hands appeared over the sheets. Her eyes were very sensitive to light now and she wore dark glasses – even the glow of the bedside lamp irritated her, and the sixty watts were replaced by forty and then draped with a cloth.

She tried reading. I bought her Stephen King's *Firestarter* in hardback, which was a mistake – it was the size of a small wardrobe and she couldn't hold it, so I rigged up a somewhat Heath Robinson affair out of a wooden tray and an old letter rack. It was not a success. One jog with her knee and it would take off across the bed like a toboggan, and I was forever on my knees trying to persuade it to come out from under the dressing table.

It was much easier for her to watch films, and I

would pick them up from the Family Video shop. At first we started out with a list headed 'Films to Watch', a selection based on reviews and personal recommendation, but as she began to consume them with an ever-increasing hunger the process degenerated into a desperate search for anything that might ease away another ninety minutes.

The staff at the shop were wonderful. They would make suggestions.

'What about . . . ?'

'She's seen it.'

'Right, well what about . . . ?'

'She's seen it.'

We could go on like that for an hour, but every now and then they would come up with a pearl that I wouldn't even have considered. More often than not, however, it was a case of:

'Well – what did she think?'

'She'd seen it.'

I began to take them home in bundles of five in the hope that just one might be a newcomer. Eventually the other customers took an interest, and I was offered advice on all sides.

'Has she seen *Mary Poppins*?'

'She's not that ill.'

'What about this, then?' asked another. He held a box in front of my face. The picture on the cover was that of a naked woman being cut in half with a chain-saw.

'I don't think so.'

'It's terrific – what it's about is, he can't stand women, you see – well, not women like that. So – he decides to rid the town of 'em and he cuts their heads off with this chain-saw. They don't hold anything back – there's blood everywhere, he kills hundreds of 'em.' He paused for effect – to let it sink in. 'They get him in the end, though.' He seemed to feel that this was an unhappy ending. 'The cops corner him and riddle him with bullets and he drops the chain-saw, but it's still going and, as he lies there helpless, it creeps along the floor and chops him to bits. It starts on his legs . . .'

'I really don't think it's her cup of tea,' I butted in. 'I really don't.' I didn't want to hurt his feelings, but he must have seen the look on my face.

'Mind you,' he said, 'there's a lot of humour in it and it's all done very tastefully.'

We watched *Starman*, I think it was, as I massaged Diana's hands. Jeff Bridges was visiting earth and we hoped that no harm would come to him – he was one of your more pleasant aliens and he had taken up with this gutsy young lady and they were on the run.

We settled back – this was promising. I put her right hand back into its cradle and started on the left. I stroked more than massaged, stroking my fingers against her palm, and then worked down the inside length of her fingers. It took about half an hour a hand – at first her fingers would be clawed and I would gently have to ease my fingertips under her

245

nails to work on the first set of knuckles. Gradually her fingers would relax as I eased my way along them, and after twenty minutes or so her hand would be halfway open. After half an hour I should be able to place my palm against her palm – her fingertips against mine. This nightly performance brought her some comfort – even though the effects wore off in an hour or so – and it made sure the hands didn't seize up completely.

It was going well, and over in America Jeff Bridges was eating his first hamburger on earth when he noticed a deer strapped over the bonnet of a hunter's car. He made his way out into the car park and we saw that the deer was dead. We watched as he laid his hands upon it, and then it kicked and broke free and ran into the forest.

'I wonder if he could do that for me?' asked Diana as I rubbed at the second set of knuckles. She had always had long fingers, but now they had lost so much muscle that they looked even longer and it was difficult to feel any padding at all.

I was almost through and then there was a gentle crack. We looked down at her hand. I'd broken her finger – her ring finger – just like that.

'I think you've broken my finger.'

'I know I have – I heard it snap.'

'How strange.'

'I was only stroking it.'

'I know.'

We stared at her hand. I can't explain the awful

feeling of having broken another's bone. It's – unexplainable. And yet she was so calm that I half expected her to say, 'Don't worry – I never liked it, an aunt gave it to me.'

'I'm sorry – does it hurt?'

'Everything hurts.'

'What shall we do?'

'To hell with it – I'm losing track of this film. Who's that man in the tartan jacket?'

Jeff Bridges made it back to his planet, and we made it over to the Hand Clinic at the Hallamshire first thing next morning. The doctor examined my handiwork closely, and then concentrated his attention on her little finger.

'This one's seizing up as well – I'm going to have to try and straighten it.'

He took the finger and bent it back. There was a crack and Diana yelled: 'You've broken it!'

'We couldn't leave it like that,' he said. Looking up at me he added, 'Try straightening them every night – they must be kept supple.'

I had been doing exactly that every night for three years or more, but now it was going to take on a new dimension.

Diana told him about her toes. They had stopped playing about and were beginning to curl under her feet. He handled them very gently but I still had to look away, half expecting a crack at any minute.

'Have a word with Fred – see if he can make something to keep them straight.'

'What on earth's causing it?'

'I haven't the slightest idea.'

Diana left the Plaster Room with trendy new hands and feet moulded from Orthoplast, a lightweight plastic material in racing white, peppered with holes to allow the skin to breathe.

'Just wear the feet at night,' Fred had told her. 'That should be enough to keep the toes straight.' Since his wonderful new creations covered the soles of her feet and then swept up into a platform for her toes, this was something of a relief.

It was a warm night that night and Diana lay on top of the sheets. She had selected the black nightdress with the lace bodice, this being a Wednesday – the straps were shoestring-thin and the skirt was slashed to the thigh. Her hair was flicked back and the blonde highlights sparkled in the gleam of a forty-watt bulb.

Her hands were encased in brilliant white Orthoplast, whilst two plastered fingers stuck out independently in an obscene gesture. Her feet stood erect, a monument to Fred's orthoplastic art and a living tribute to Popeye's Olive Oil.

She examined her reflection in the dressing-table mirror.

'I look ridiculous.'

'No, you don't.'

'I don't know whether to commit suicide or run away and join a circus.'

I laughed and she laughed with me. Then, propping herself up on her elbows, she studied her reflection closely and turned sad eyes upon me.

'It's not really funny, is it?'

The rebellious toes brought her spirits crashing. The devices on her hands were old hat now – she could perform small miracles of dexterity whilst wearing them, and it almost seemed that she had always worn them – but the very act of strapping her feet at night indicated that there was more to come and brought her tumbling down at the end of the day.

Every now and then she would leave them off, but then the toes would bunch and it would be impossible for her to wear shoes or for me to walk her across the room.

It's bloody hard to lift someone when they have every reason to be depressed. It's much easier to join them in their depression and wallow there together. So I wallowed – not a big wallow, I just dipped my toe in the edge for a day and, thus recharged, set about building her up again. I was usually pretty good at that. A letter from the BBC, a commission from a magazine or a smile from a passing Jack Russell would fill me with such soaring optimism that it would overflow and wash over Diana. But this time I was getting nowhere. She buried herself within herself and spent hours lying on her side, staring at the curtains.

I tried everything from the sublime to the ridiculous. A dozen roses: 'Very nice – thank you.' The long, heartfelt monologue on how things could be worse, how at least we had each other and how our love would conquer all: 'I suppose so.' The shock tactic of quoting the vicar in Lewis's lift. 'You should be thankful, my dear, that God has chosen you.' This usually had her spitting fire, but she just gave a thin smile and disappeared under the sheets.

The trouble was I tried too hard. I held her close and talked logically and sensibly – so sensibly and logically that I spent the rest of the day lost in admiration for myself. I applied transfers of Garfield to the slabs of Orthoplast on her feet so that she would see them when she woke – and later spent an hour scrubbing off his grinning image in the sink.

But she was on to me and she was having none of it. This threw me into a deep depression, and she rallied slightly as she tried to cheer me up.

I was attempting to do something interesting with a rollmop when Nick and Jo called to talk about the wedding. I enjoyed the odd rollmop but I found them so disgusting that I had to eat them with my eyes shut and I thought a sandwich might do the trick.

'Have you seen my fishing rod?' Nick wanted to know.

'You haven't got a fishing rod.'

Jo agreed with me. 'I didn't think he had a fishing rod.'

I agreed with Jo. 'He doesn't have a fishing rod.'

'It was a wooden one that split into three parts, with a thing you wind on one end and a nylon line with a hook on the other.'

I had to admit that it sounded very much like a fishing rod – in fact I couldn't think of anything else it could have been, but I knew damn well that he had never owned a fishing rod in his life.

'You don't go fishing,' Jo told him.

'I don't now – but I did then.'

'When?' I asked.

'At Westward Ho.'

'Good grief! You were only seven when we went to Westward Ho.'

'But I did have a fishing rod. You haven't sold it, have you? You're always selling my things.'

I was quite stunned. 'I have never sold any of your things,' I told him. 'You tell me when I ever sold any of your things.'

'This week you have sold my bed, my wardrobe, my bookcase and my big cupboard.'

'That's true,' I admitted, 'but apart from that – you tell me when I ever sold any of your things.'

'Isn't that enough?' he said, loping off upstairs to see his mother. 'She'll know where my fishing rod is.'

I turned to Jo. 'I've only taken a deposit on them. He said you wouldn't need them in the new house, and I want his room for an office.'

'I know,' she said, and gave me a kiss. I rather liked the thought of having a daughter-in-law. 'Has he got a fishing rod?'

'No – it must be fifteen years since we went to Westward Ho. He had a rod then, but I only hired it for the week.'

Nick sauntered into the kitchen carrying a device that split into three sections. The thickest section had a cork handle with a thing you wind fastened to it, while the other two sections were slightly tapered and bore rings to restrain a nylon line. Only the hook appeared to be missing.

'That,' he said, 'is a fishing rod.'

'Where did you find it?'

'Mum knew where it was – in the loft with your snorkel and flippers.'

'I mean originally.'

'It's the one you bought me in Westward Ho.'

I couldn't believe it. 'I didn't *buy* it for you – I hired it at three and six a week. You weren't supposed to bring it home.'

'How was I to know?'

This was ridiculous. Diana had been able to tell him exactly where to put his hands on a fishing rod that hadn't seen the light of day for fifteen years. Yet not twelve months ago she had denied all knowledge of my snorkel and flippers.

'One hundred and thirty-six pounds ten shillings,' said Jo.

'Pardon?'

'That's what you owe the man in Westward Ho at three and six a week for fifteen years. One hundred and thirty-six pounds and ten shillings.'

Not only did I have a future daughter-in-law who would give me a hug and a kiss now and then, but she could also add up in real money. I was most impressed.

They went upstairs to talk about the wedding, and I went off to the studio to record a piece on the mating habits of the wild strawberry.

When I returned they were on their way downstairs and ready to leave.

'How's your mum?'

'She's fine.'

She always could put on a show, and she wouldn't want Jo to see how depressed she felt.

'Nick – why all the sudden interest in fishing?'

'We're going to a car boot sale on Sunday – I'm rounding up anything there is to sell.'

They needed every penny they could lay their hands on, what with the new house and the wedding.

'You can have my snorkel and flippers, if that's any help.'

'Thanks – I've put them in the car already. Mum said it would be all right.'

★

I made two coffees and, pausing at the bedroom door, put on my 'Everything's all right with the world' smile and sailed on in.

She was lying in the dark and for a moment I thought she was asleep. Then a tired voice said, 'Hullo.'

'Hullo – are you all right?' I sat on the edge of the bed. 'I've brought you a coffee.

'I don't think I can move at the moment – sorry.'

'It doesn't matter.'

'I'm going to need a bath before I can sleep.'

'OK.'

I put the coffee on the table and lay down beside her in the dark and touched her arm.

'That hurts – sorry.'

'I didn't think.'

She moved slightly to be facing me and put her head against my shoulder.

'I've been a wimp.'

'No, you haven't.'

'Yes, I have, and you've tried everything to get me out of it.'

'I did my best.'

'You've been an absolute pain in the arse.'

'Thank you.'

'But it's all over now – it's finished.'

'How do you mean?'

'I'm too tired to make a grand gesture – but I'm out of it now.' She moved on to her back. 'Tomorrow we invade Poland.'

She slept then, and I set up my typewriter on the dining table downstairs and dreamed of the day, very soon now, when I would convert Nick's bedroom into an office.

An hour or so later she signalled me. It was a sophisticated system that we had rigged up – I would position her elbow crutch on the edge of the bed and, when she woke, one raised knee would send it crashing to the floor.

As I bathed her, the pain subsided and she came to life.

'Listening to Nick and Jo talk about the wedding did it – it's been depressing me that I couldn't do anything for them.'

'Everyone understands.'

'Do you remember that little nurse at the Maudsley?'

'The wiry one?'

'Yes – she asked me if you shouted at me.'

'She asked me that as well.'

'I told her you didn't.'

'I don't.' I sponged her shoulders and then she lay back and soaked.

'I've told Nick and Jo that I'll make all the bridesmaids' dresses for them.'

'You what?'

'Don't shout.'

'You can't, love – it's not possible.'

'I can and I will. I'm sure the girls at the embroidery class will help me – I know I can do it.'

I wrapped her in a towel and lifted her from the bath. She sat on the stool and I dried her. She was a trier – she would make the dresses somehow, but at what cost?

She looked so tired and worn out as I carried her to the bedroom. I eased her fingers into Fred's hands and then set about her feet. The toes had curled, and I had to massage each one before I could force them down on the plastic platforms.

It was a warm night and we slept naked with just a sheet over us. Down at the bottom of the bed her feet stood guard – erect like two small ghosts.

She looked over the sheet and examined them.

'Tell you something else.'

'What's that?'

'To hell with the wheelchair – I'm going to walk down that bloody aisle.'

17

I hauled the kitten out of the tumble dryer and dropped it back over the fence. I had been about to switch the machine on when I noticed a little white furry thing stamping all over the washing, and for a brief moment I was tempted to give him the ride of his life. This was the third time in as many weeks I had found his dirty great hoof prints all over the pillow cases, and he was fast becoming public enemy number one – a marked kitten.

A week ago I had been driving over to Derby. The sun was shining and the radio playing and I was just passing through Belper when something tapped me on the shoulder. I almost drove straight through the front door of a pub, and when I glanced in the driving mirror there was this kitten, front paws on my shoulder, grinning at me in my own mirror. I locked him in the car in Derby and was told off by a large lady traffic warden for not leaving a window open.

'He could suffocate.'

'I'm banking on it.'

It was a very weird kitten. Diana had been the first to catch sight of him.

'There's a very tall kitten moved in across the road.'

I had never thought of kittens being very tall, or very short for that matter.

'How tall?'

'Just an ordinary kitten on stilts – a white one.'

'Oh, I've seen him,' Sally had remarked, 'peering over the car.'

'He can't be as tall as all that.'

Apparently he had been standing on the fence at the time and so there was no immediate need for me to run screaming into the streets, but he was a remarkable kitten – he had built-up paws. He sat on the carport and planned his next offensive as I reversed the car out of the garage and drove down to Orchard House.

Diana had set about the bridesmaids' dresses with an enthusiasm that carried her through the initial stages, but now the sewing machine had defeated her. The wire cages prevented her from moving the fabric around freely, and when she had tried to work without them the fingers had quickly clawed.

Her foot wouldn't come off the pedal when she told it to, and the frustrations were building up. She had tried beating the sewing machine with a hair-brush, but it had little effect and the snide references to its parentage served only to make it even more sullen and broody than before.

She had cut out the smallest dress for the mini-bridesmaid and begun to sew it up, but it was a slow, laborious business – ten minutes on, two hours off – and apart from the exhaustion and the pain she couldn't focus her eyes, or her mind, for long. I would tuck her up in bed where she could shut out the disappointment and sleep.

And so we had called in reinforcements. Down at Orchard House Joyce Murray had opened her home and set up a production unit. Around an enormous table sat Louise and Leslie, Margaret and Val, Gill and Joyce herself, cutting and trimming and drinking huge quantities of tea. Diana, more often than not, lay on a settee, hand-sewing all day until the pain took over and the sweat ran down her face.

Those days at Orchard House were some of the happiest days of her life. Often she could only lie on the settee and watch, the non-playing captain urging on her team from the pavilion. That so many friends should want to help and take so much pleasure in the task was rewarding and exhilarating – and it was knocking the stuffing out of her.

Meanwhile the men of the family had important business to conduct. We were to wear tails at the wedding – blue ones. The ushers would be in grey, but the key personnel – the groom, best man, bride's father and me – were to be kitted out in blue-striped trousers and waistcoat, dark blue jacket and a topper.

The waistcoat was like no waistcoat I had ever seen – just two pieces that buttoned up the front and no back. There were two strings of elastic around the neck and the waist, but I could cut those off later. The coat and trousers fitted me like a glove, but it was when I tried on the top hat that the outfit came alive. There was no doubt about it – I was born to wear a top hat. Either you can or you can't, and I could – maybe it had something to do with my military bearing, with my father having been in the Fire Service.

I stepped out of the cubicle and into the shop and the assistant in charge of my case immediately stepped forward, took off my hat and replaced it the other way round.

'You had it on back to front,' he told me.

I looked in the mirror – it had looked better back to front.

'There's still something not quite right.'

'Will you be wearing the Kajagoogoo tee-shirt on the day, sir?'

'You know about these things – what do you think?'

He thought not – it would detract from the solemnity of the occasion. It would have been wasted anyway - both the 'Kaj' and the final 'goo' would have been hidden by the waistcoat.

In between bouts at Orchard House Diana rested. This was serious resting, none of your dilettante stuff. She was going to walk down that aisle and so she worked at it as seriously as a boxer in training. Stress was kept down to a minimum and a high-fibre diet was introduced into the scheme of things until a bowl of gravel would have been a delicacy. Vitamins were pumped into her until she rattled.

The only negative element to creep past the guards was the belated report from the Maudsley. Dr MacFarlane was a positive force, but even he couldn't read anything into the report that might set the pulses racing.

'Do they think it's all in my mind?'

'Not really – they just . . . er . . . . Not really.'

He had helped her through some sticky patches on this particular wicket, and he was finding it harder and harder to know where to go next.

'I have an idea, a hospital in London – I'll make some enquiries.'

'No more hospitals.'

'I'll get back to you.'

She took the report badly. The tests had proved nothing, and once again the veiled suggestion that she was just another hysterical woman had been raised. She moved through anger to tears and back again. She talked until the small hours, reliving the many interviews with those who doubted that she had anything wrong with her at all – anything, that is, that had not been induced by an over-active imagination.

At first she had quite enjoyed the inevitable question, 'How's your sex life?' She could even bring a blush from the younger doctors with – 'Fine – how's yours?' But now it had taken on a more

sinister connotation, as had, 'The mind plays peculiar tricks, you know.' This was usually followed
by, 'I could give you some tranquillizers.'

The menopause played a large part in this 'We-
can't-find-anything-and-we're-never-wrong – so-
you-must-be-imagining-it' theory.

'Have you been through the menopause?'

'I don't know. I've been so bloody ill these past
few years. I sweat buckets – I could have missed it.'

Gradually the anger worked its way out of her
system, as anger must, and the wedding prepara-
tions took over.

'I shall have to buy a hat.'

She had never worn a hat since the day we left for
Shanklin on our honeymoon.

'I look silly in hats.'

The old photographs of our honeymoon tended
to confirm this point of view, and the evidence
mounted as we combed the millinery mines of
Sheffield.

'Let's try Coles,' I suggested. I knew nothing
about hats, but they had a licensed restaurant and it
was calling to me. As I pushed the wheelchair along
a narrow side street we came across a small shop,
and in the window were half a dozen hats mounted
on chrome stalks.

'Let's try in there.'

'Let's go to Coles first – we can try there on the
way back,' and we sailed on past.

The body in the wheelchair before me stiffened

262

and the hands moved towards the brakes. I'd done it again – it's so easy to have the final word when you are dealing with the back of a head. No consultation – you just keep on pushing.

'Sorry.' I wheeled the chair around and we squeezed in through the hat shop door.

It proved a fruitless excursion but, with honour satisfied, we were able to smile at one another above the menus as the waitress hovered.

'How does she like her steak, sir?'

'Rare.'

'Would she prefer potatoes or chips?'

'Potatoes, I think.'

No point in fighting back. She was a nice girl and she was trying desperately hard not to stare at Diana's hands.

'You didn't tell her about my periods.'

'Thought I'd save it for the sweet.'

The chair nosed its way through winter coats, skirted the Windsmoor ghetto and there before us, just beyond the double-knits, lay the long-lost valley of hats. I have never seen so many feathers in my life – small round mirrors were angled down to wheelchair level as hat after hat was plonked on the small round head.

The first fifteen hundred or so did nothing for her but the assistant persevered until – 'What about this one?'

It was red, with feathers and a veil, and it had

been designed especially for Diana by Bill Horsman. I had never heard of Bill, but he obviously knew Diana very well.

'That's it – that's the one.'

We snorted at the models in the little shop as we trundled past on our way back to the car.

'Pathetic,' muttered Diana, clutching her carrier bag to her breast and then hoisting it high above her head as though it were the FA cup.

As we left the car park she dived in amongst the tissue paper and took out the hat. Placing it on her head, she pulled down the mirror and for some time looked at herself in silence.

'I look beautiful.'

'You do – very beautiful.'

'I know.'

And then, tipping the hat forward so that it wouldn't be crushed by the headrest, she fell asleep – the little white price ticket dangling against her nose.

Ian Hunt was to be Nick's best man, and he was to be found more often than not rehearsing his speech in our kitchen. The clean bits changed daily, but the rude bits remained – it was a good job my mother was going deaf.

Ian worried constantly about his speech. He was built like a brick out-house and nobody in their right mind would tell him that it was anything but brilliant, but still he worried.

Nick worried about his speech and did nothing about it until the morning of the wedding.

'Right, Dad – what are we going to do about this speech, then?'

'What do you mean – we?'

'Come on, you love deadlines.'

I pulled out the typewriter and together we rattled off a passable oration whilst Ian paced up and down behind us, rehearsing and cutting and adding yet more rude bits. Then Nick went up for a bath and I polished his speech until it shone whilst Ian lay on the hearthrug in a coma.

I handed the two sheets of paper to Nick as we passed on the stairs. 'Yes – I can do something with that. Thanks, Dad – just needs polishing.'

My mother was discussing the catering arrangements with Whisky as I arrived to pick her up. Three dishes were lined up in front of a somewhat bemused cat, each one covered with a check gingham bonnet. She took him on a tour of the line, explaining to him as she went.

'This one's your lunch – that one's your supper – that one's a snack in case you get hungry – and there's two toffees, but you're not to spoil your appetite – I've unwrapped them for you.'

The cat looked in disbelief – at least he wouldn't have to unwrap the toffees. He moved in on the third dish and began to wrestle with the gingham cover.

'Not that one – that's your supper.' She picked him up and plonked him down in front of his lunch. 'That one.'

She whipped off the cover for him and he plunged his head deep into the dish. He ate steadily for a minute or two and then sat back, a faraway look in his eyes – the contents seemed undisturbed. I leaned forward and peeled away the clingfilm stretched tight across the top of the dish, and he nodded to me and tried once more.

'What is that – tuna?'

'Pilchards – he loves pilchards.'

'What's he having for his supper?'

'Pilchards – he loves them, he's gone right off rabbit.'

'What about the snack?'

'Pilchards.'

I thought about it for a moment or so. 'Why does he have to eat them in any particular order, then?'

'He can't go having his supper before his lunch.'

I should have thought it out more carefully – I was always making a fool of myself – and so I waited a while before I asked.

'Are the other two dishes covered with clingfilm?'

'Course – it keeps them lovely and fresh.'

'He can't get it off.'

'I'll take it off – at the very last minute.'

She put the final touches to her make-up, switched on the television for Whisky and then switched off the electricity at the mains.

'Right – are you ready?'

'Yes.'

'Let's go.'

She whipped off the clingfilm, slammed down the covers and we raced for the door, leaving Whisky gaping in our wake.

We had hidden the wheelchair by the side of the church. It was a pity in a way – Sally had decorated it with silk flowers and streamers and it looked a treat. It would be produced later on, but for the time being Diana was standing by the church door, wedged between brother-in-law Harry and me. She seemed to have peaked at just the right time; she was happy and excited and running on pure adrenalin.

The churchyard was crowded with jostling friends and relatives as we waited for the bride to arrive. My mother, in her splendid light blue and navy hat, fresh from the Co-op, chatted happily to people she had never met and was surprised how much they knew about her.

'Where did you hear about that?'

'Deric mentioned it on the radio.'

'Did he?' She moved towards me to find out why I should have mentioned her aversion to duvets on the radio, and what was this I had been saying about her being addicted to buttercup syrup. Fortunately she was sidetracked by another admirer, and as the afternoon wore on she developed quite a taste for the limelight.

The bride was due at any time, and Mrs Henshaw was just wondering where Nick and Ian had got to when the pair of them came sauntering down from the Duke William, toppers in hand, as though they did this every Saturday afternoon.

It was time for us to file into church. Diana gritted her teeth and off we set. We had practised at home with my arm around her waist and my left hand under her elbow, but we hadn't reckoned on the top hat.

I held it between forefinger and thumb, and it dangled at such an angle that everyone could see the contents. My cigarettes and lighter, the best man's cigarettes and lighter and the chief usher's cigarettes and lighter.

Together with these tobacconist's sundries were two boxes of confetti, a hand support that was not to be seen on the photographs, two Heinz beans cans tied together with a piece of string, the front door key of Nick's house, three rolls of film from a Minolta camera and two fag ends, the property of Jo's youngest brother Mark, in case his mother frisked him during the ceremony.

The hired suits had no pockets, and so the top hat became as indispensable as a wire basket in a super-market.

Diana made it – she buckled slightly at the furlong mark, but she made it and fell into the front pew with a happy smile on her face.

The bride looked stunning and the service went

like a dream – in the vestry afterwards Diana faced the long trek back, this time on the arm of the bride's father.

Geoff had it all worked out. Jo's brother Andrew took one elbow and Geoff the other. They moved elegantly and smoothly, and at no point throughout the journey did Diana's feet touch the floor.

It was a lovely day and Diana sailed through it on a high. The speeches went well, rude bits and all, and my mother laughed throughout, despite only hearing the odd word in ten. She drank her champagne well before the toasts and then calmly pinched a glass from the person on her left.

The person on her left was Rosie's son Robert, who was too polite and too small to argue.

'Are you Deric or Diana's mother?'

Now this sort of technical question is liable to throw her completely and she needed time to consider her response.

'Er . . . ' she gazed with furrowed brow at the little boy. 'I'm . . . er . . . er . . . ' and then her face brightened. 'I'm Deric's father,' she declared, and that out of the way she reached over and pinched Rosie's wine as well.

That night we lay in bed and talked the day to pieces until Diana could talk no more. As she slept, my thoughts turned to more practical matters – I had lost a son and gained an office. I would have the desk by the window and shelves all along the wall – a wooden filing cabinet, not metal, and that swivel chair so that I could swing round and fix visitors with a steely eye after shouting, 'Come!' Early next morning, six-thirty on the dot, I was out of bed and measuring.

Diana got out of bed three and half months later just in time for New Year's Eve.

I had been down to the studio and as I crept up the stairs, so as not to waken her, I heard the sound of the television. I pushed the door open gently and looked in.

Her fingers were spread on the sheet before her and the freshly painted nails were laid out to dry. Her feet peeped out from under the turned-back blanket, a tiny red blob decorating the end of each and every curly toe.

She wore a scarlet nightdress – the 'upper-class tart' model that my mother had bought her – and perched bravely on her head was the little red hat.

She heard me and turned towards the door, beaming at me through the veil.

'I shall wear this hat at my funeral.'

'While we all sing "Wide Eyed and Legless"?'

'Yes.'

Mavis Nicholson was taking a deep breath, and Diana zapped her before she could launch her next question into space.

'I thought it might add a touch of class to the proceedings.'

I didn't want to hear any more about funerals. Selfishly I couldn't bear the thought of losing her. She rounded off my life – without her it would be all sharp corners.

'Pity I missed Christmas again.'

'You didn't miss much – it was a very quiet affair. Next year we'll go away and be spoilt.'

'I don't think I shall see another.'

'Don't be silly. There's nothing wrong with you anyway – it's all in your head.'

'That's true.' She examined the painted nails through her veil and then smiled up at me. 'Happy New Year.'

'Happy New Year, love – fancy a cup of coffee?'

'I'd love one, and Deric . . .'

'Yes?'

'Promise you won't forget about the hat.'

18

I was beginning to get suspicious. David and Joyce were upright, solid citizens and yet they were lying in their teeth.

'Diana can't come to the phone at the moment, Deric – Joyce is giving her a bath.'

'She's just having a lie-down, Deric. It's been a busy day – David took us down to the beach.'

She seemed to be having one hell of a weekend. I had phoned the Isle of Wight twice a day from the Earnley Concourse just outside Chichester, and on each occasion Diana was unable to take the call.

'She's not well, is she, Joyce? Be honest with me.'

'She's fine. She's just having a sleep. She's been . . .'

'Scuba diving?'

'No . . .'

'Rock climbing?'

'No . . . she's fine, honest.'

She hadn't been fine on the way down. She had blacked out in a café just off the A34, and again in Southsea as we waited for the hovercraft.

'You can't go across on your own.'

'I shall hardly be on my own.' She indicated the

gathering crowd of passengers. 'And Joyce and David will be waiting for me.'

When Joyce and David had heard at Nick's wedding that I had been invited to a writers' weekend in Chichester they immediately offered Diana a weekend in Freshwater.

'Joyce is a nurse – she'll look after me.'

I didn't doubt it for one moment, but the journey down had done her no good at all and the pain had been such that just outside Oxford we had taken a motel bedroom for a couple of hours so that Diana could rest up. The receptionist had winked and told me that lots of couples booked in for just an hour or so.

As the hovercraft frisbied up the ramp we were joined by a polio victim from Rotherham. He was lying on what looked like a converted tea trolley and he could move his head, but nothing else – so he nodded.

The two of them were trundled on board by the ferry staff, who did everything right and parked them in the aisle under a large sign that read: 'In case of accident, your lifebelt is on the back of your seat.'

'If we have an accident – are you going to get my lifebelt or shall I get yours?' Diana asked him.

In the end they decided they would probably both drown, and on that happy note I kissed her goodbye and set off for Chichester.

The Earnley Concourse was a delight, and I met old friends and new friends including P. D. James.

'Have you always been interested in murder?'

'When I was five I read Humpty Dumpty and I thought – did he fall or was he pushed?'

Peacocks decorate the lawns at Earnley and have orgasms outside your bedroom window at six o'clock in the morning. One bird in particular would have been strangled by my bare hands even though it was the size of a small ostrich, but the risk of being unmasked as the killer by P. D. James was far too great.

Joyce and David had met the hovercraft and whipped Diana off to their bungalow by the sea. An hour later she had collapsed and spent the three days in bed – fortunately they had left the window open, and so she was able to smell the sea if the breeze was in the right direction.

It was Tuesday before she was well enough to travel and Joyce wanted a word with me before we left.

'I had no idea she was so ill.'

'She puts on a good act.'

'On Monday I got her into the bathroom and left her for a moment. When I returned she'd had a blackout and her head was in the washbasin. It was empty – but it doesn't bear thinking about.'

The two of them had been wonderful, and they had lied to me over the phone as though they had been doing it all their lives.

'Diana made us do it – she's very forceful.'

'Don't I know it.'

As we pulled on to the M1, Diana told me how much she had enjoyed the weekend.

'It was a lovely bedroom.'

I couldn't understand why we were on the M1 – navigation isn't my strong point – but just a few miles south of Watford Gap the pain flooded out of her.

'Let's go in there.'

There was the Blue Boar Service Station, and we tackled a cup of tea and a cheese sandwich.

'Do I look brown?'

'Very brown.'

'Must have been the sea air.'

She smiled around her at the harassed salesmen and the child-worn trippers, and admired the plastic flowers slung from the ceiling.

'It was worth coming,' she said, 'just for this cheese sandwich.'

It took a month before the exhaustion allowed her to crawl out of bed under her own steam – God knows how long it would have taken if there had been anything wrong with her.

This time, however, her spirit didn't bounce back in tandem. Whilst in the past the long line of specialists had failed to put a name to her condition, there would always be another, tucked away in some hospital, who would take one look at her and say, 'I once saw something similar to this in Burma during the war.'

The hope had been a slender one, but it had been there. Now she had done with hospitals, no more disappointments – but also no odd flash of fleeting optimism, and without it life was heading downhill.

We had often thought of calling Dr Patrick Harvey. He had stayed in our thoughts ever since that day he came to check out Diana's claim for the invalidity pension and attendance allowance. He had listened to her then and he seemed to under-stand – he wasn't in the business of defending the system against all-comers.

He understood that Diana wasn't about to throw bricks because the specialists couldn't work miracles – that she didn't expect miracles, but that she just wanted to be part of a team that would search for a cause, for a reason why her body was falling apart. That all she wanted was to be taken seriously and not labelled as a hysterical woman simply because there wasn't an entry in the book for her particular collection of ills.

He understood this, but above all he had lis-tened, and that is a rare quality in the National Health Service where specialists tend to listen on the run and offer a Van Gogh's ear to their patients.

He had said we could ring him if Diana needed

to talk – so we rang and made an appointment, and within days I was helping her climb the staircase at his home. His office was on the first floor.

An hour later I was helping her down and into the car, and Diana was fuming.

'He was so bloody rude!'

I got it all. How he had questioned everything she had told him, how he had argued with everything she had said, how he had made her so mad that she felt like poking him in the eye with one of Fred's wire struts.

The commentary went on and on as we waded through the food hall in Marks & Spencer's, as she tried on a pair of sensible bloody shoes in Peter Lord and as we tried in vain to stuff a six-pack of toilet rolls into one of Boots's stupid little wire baskets.

She finally ran out of steam and invective as we passed Arthur Hind's farm on the way home, and the fire turned to smoke and slowly fizzled out.

'My God, he was rude!' she said as she flexed the sharp bit on her thumb protector and peeled away absently at the licence disc on the windscreen.

'He was insufferable – I'm going again on Tuesday.'

Patrick Harvey had become disillusioned with the Health Service. He now worked privately as a psychotherapist and he had achieved considerable success with incurable cancer patients, helping them come to terms with their illness.

Diana went to do battle with him once a week. He would listen to her and then she would have to listen to him. Gradually he worked away at the inner rage that boiled over at the unfairness of it all, and between them they lowered her aims and yet extended the design of her life so that, over the months, a certain calm began to flow through her – a stillness that owed nothing to acceptance, but which was born of self-knowledge.

She relaxed and stopped fighting the pain and paralysis – there was no defeat, but now she tried to tame it rather than beat it to death with a stick, and above all she was being treated as an intelligent woman, who could be pretty stupid now and then, but a woman whose grip on life was respected enough to be challenged.

This peace of mind percolated through the house, and the effect was unnerving.

'What was that crash?'

'The bathroom cabinet fell off the wall.'

'How?'

'I grabbed it when I slipped – I'll fix it.'

'Leave it – I shall be able to reach it now it's on the floor.'

Nick employed Diana as his chief strategist in moments of stress. He had taken on a new wife, a new house and a new job with Copystatic – there were problems at work.

'. . . so what do you think I should do? I can't just sit back and let them get away with it.'

'Tell me – what were you worrying about three months ago?'

'I can't remember.'

'No – and you won't remember this three months from now.'

Sally took a break from the Sheraton Park Towers Casino in London, where she was now plying her trade as a croupier.

'Is Mum on drugs?'

'A dozen or so pain killers a day.'

'Is she smoking cannabis?'

'No – why?'

'I've never known her like this.'

'She's seeing Dr Harvey once a week.'

'Can I have his telephone number?'

Even so, when Dr MacFarlane suggested a visit to yet another hospital I had a feeling that this new-found wave of serenity would smash against the rocks.

'What do you think she'll say?'

'I think she'll say no.'

'So do I.'

Still, he went upstairs to put the idea to her – and came back down again soon afterwards with a faraway look on his face.

'Well?'

'She's all for it – she thinks that this time they might find something.'

I saw him off the premises and then made a mental note to ask Sally what cannabis smelt like.

The National Hospital for Nervous Diseases in Queen Square, London is the most amazing place. Diana was to be in the new wing, which had been opened by Princess Alice of Athlone in 1937. God knows who opened the old wing – probably Richard III.

I received my instructions from the old family retainer in the main hall, and after negotiating several miles of corridor we eventually found Gower ward somewhere just north of Staines. It was lunchtime and the air was thick with disinfectant and boiled carrots.

'Let's go and have a pizza,' Diana suggested, and so I wheeled her round and we retreated. One deep pan pizza and four glasses of red wine later we returned and threw ourselves on their mercy.

The ward was like a MASH unit – the patients were battle-hardened veterans who had been around, they had served their apprenticeship in infirmaries all over the country and their days were full of pain and frustration. They knew more about their own condition than the average general practitioner, and they were not to be trifled with.

The patients in wheelchairs fetched and carried for those who were totally immobile, and those with brain damage were listened to carefully as it was understood that they were not stupid – just that it took them some time to sort the words out properly.

Amidst the chaos a nurse lay on an empty bed reading the *Daily Mirror*, conserving her energy for the moment when she would have to leap into action.

There was no suggestion that Diana should be tucked up in bed, and so we packed away her bits and pieces and sat talking together by the window until, one by one, the walking wounded came over to check us out.

'If you get anything pinched, love, it'll be her over there in the end bed.'

Her over there sat up primly in the end bed and waved to us as our eyes flicked over her.

There seemed to be a lot of cross-pollination with the men's ward around the corner, and Gareth, Peter and Richard introduced themselves.

'Before you go to the toilet get one of the male nurses to have a look first – there's cockroaches in there you could throw a saddle over.'

Gradually I was squeezed out of the inner circle as more patients came over and joined in. Then, just as the buzz of conversation reached its height, it faded as heads turned to watch *her over there in the end bed* pad quietly towards the ward door.

The nurse lowered her *Daily Mirror* and then, as the slippered figure disappeared, she leapt into action and, racing over the polished floor, broke open the locker by the door.

'Blue knickers,' she shouted, waving a pair in the air.

'Mine!'

'Twenty Silk Cut and a box of matches.'

'Over here!'

'Ronson Escort hair dryer with blue and pink flowered plastic hood.'

'Bloody hell!'

'A quarter of mint lumps.'

Silence.

'They must be hers.'

'*Playboy* magazine.'

Silence again and then, 'I know whose that is – I'll take it for him.'

'Powder compact – brown.'

'Here!'

'Lipstick – Mary Quant.'

' . . . and again.'

The inventory went on and on until a signal from the guard told us that someone was approaching. The nurse flung herself back behind her *Daily Mirror* and the ward looked on as *her over there in the end bed* padded back in and sat down.

With a smile of pure joy on her face she reached under her dressing gown and produced two toilet rolls and a bottle of Izal liquid, and after stroking each lovingly in turn she tucked them safely away in the back of her locker.

Diana smiled up at me, 'I think I'm going to like it here,' she said.

Sally was working in the casino that afternoon and I had arranged to meet her in the hospital that evening – around eight-thirty, she had said, but there was no sign of her as I walked into the ward.

There was no sign of Diana either. A large bouquet stood on her bedside locker, but her bed was empty and I plonked my grapes under the flowers and read the Interflora card: 'Diana Longden. The National Hospital for Mental Disorders – with love from Sally.'

The owner of the Mary Quant lipstick shouted across at me: 'She's gone to the pub, darling, with Gareth and Richard and a young lady in a short skirt.'

I found the sister, who confirmed the diagnosis. She had just returned from a cockroach hunt and was scraping the soles of her shoes against a radiator.

'That's right, she's nipped out for a drink – I've told them to be back for ten-thirty. She said for you to meet them there.'

'Right – what's the name of the pub?'

'Now that she didn't say.'

I combed every pub in Queen Square, Boswell Street and Old Gloucester Street before I gave up and sat waiting on the steps outside the hospital. An old man sitting by my side offered me a swig of his meths, which was nice of him, but I wasn't thirsty. He had lived in Coventry up until a year ago, but he had come down to London because that's where the opportunities were these days.

Out of the gloom a wheelchair appeared, swerving across the square at high speed, with Diana aboard and either Richard or Gareth pushing. Not far behind, in second place, came Sally pushing either Gareth or Richard.

'We found this grotty wine bar – it was great,' Diana enthused.

'Mum blacked out twice,' Sally told me, 'but lots of customers had passed out so nobody took any notice.'

The old man looked up – sounded interesting, this place.

Later Diana and I said our goodbyes – it was going to be a long stay this time, but I would be down at the weekends and Sally was only a tube ride away. The flowers were still standing proudly on the bedside locker, but the grapes had disappeared and sucking and spitting noises were coming from the end bed as Sally and I pushed our way through the door.

'Did you know you addressed the bouquet to "The National Hospital for Mental Disorders"?'

'What should it be?'

'Nervous Diseases.'

'Oh, hell!'

The old man danced a little jig for us as we left the hospital, and then raised his bottle in salute as a nurse struggled up the steps dragging an enormous green rabbit behind her. Being a gentleman he propped open the door and then took the front legs as she took the back legs and together they man-handled it into the building.

Who knows? Maybe Sally had the address right after all.

I rang the hospital twice a day, morning and even-ing, and received regular bulletins from Sally. At home it was Diana's eyes that told me exactly how she was feeling – on the phone her voice gave the game away.

Sometimes she was too ill to talk to me and I would have to wait for Sally's report.

'She's fine – she's just gone down to X-ray.'

'She was down there this morning when I rang.'

'Yes – well, she's down there again.'

'Why?'

'She told me not to tell you.'

'Tell me or I shall hit you.'

'She was showing one of the boys how she could do a wheelie on two wheels round the corner and she forgot about the slippery floor and the wheel-chair turned over and they think she's broken her ankle.'

This was a trick she had perfected in the early days – she would persuade someone to give her a push, gather up a head of steam and then let go. As she approached the corner she would throw her weight over to one side and fly round on two wheels. It was most dramatic, and she had perfected the trick whilst watching Barry Sheene on television – I had told her what had happened to Barry Sheene, and she had told me that he didn't have her experience.

'Mum says it's the leg that doesn't work, anyway, so we're not to worry.'

I told the story that night at a massed meeting of Women's Institutes where I was guest speaker – it didn't go down well. The consensus of opinion seemed to swing between, 'What a silly thing to do,' and 'Oh, the poor woman.'

My mother got it right when I told her the next morning as she washed the cat in the kitchen sink. She listened to every word and then said, 'She's a bugger, isn't she – but you have to hand it to her.'

My third weekend in London was a low-key affair. There were no pints and pizzas this time – Diana was too ill even to talk at any length, and the staff were both puzzled and alarmed. This was a very different woman from the one who had introduced the turbo-charged wheelchair to the ward.

The broken ankle was a minor irritant compared with the constant blackouts, the violent headaches and the raging temperature. Then, when it seemed she could take no more, the hands began to claw and twist. I called the sister and we dealt with it as best we could. In effect we watched her suffer and I said things like, 'It's all right, love – I'm with you,' and tried to convince myself that it helped.

The weekend was one of silent apology – of reproach for being healthy and for not being able to do a damn thing for her. A weekend of silent loving and of words that turned into platitudes the moment they escaped. It was a long weekend – it lasted for two whole days, and then Sally took over on the Monday and I went home.

I was knackered, both physically and emotionally, but I set the alarm for six-thirty next morning – you have no right to be knackered when you are fit and well. I slept through until three forty-five in the afternoon and rang the hospital in a panic before I was awake. Sally took the call eventually, and held the phone so that Diana could tell me herself how much better she was.

'I've just eaten some liver.'

'Fish,' I heard Sally whisper.

'We think it could have been fish – so you don't have to worry now, do you?'

The gales had whipped Matlock in my absence, and the garden looked as though gypsies had recently upped their caravans and left. First of all I picked the fence up off the lawn and placed it back between us and them next door where God had intended it should be, and then I went in search of the dustbin.

It had wrapped itself round the base of the cherry tree and disgorged its contents all over the lawn and rockery. The tall kitten from across the road was dribbling the cap from an HP sauce bottle in and out of the teabags. A solid tackle from behind was enough to dispossess him, and he transferred his attention to a solid ingot of yellow custard that was lying on its back, sunning itself on the lawn. I had no idea that one family could work its way through so many teabags in a single week and, after picking up several hundred, tentatively between finger and thumb, I began heeling them in on the assumption that I might be putting some goodness back into the earth.

It was the hard-boiled egg from under Nick's bed that gave me the inspiration. It was sitting up nicely on a tuft of grass just by the black cherry yoghurt carton, and so I fetched my golf clubs out of the car and a five iron dispatched it neatly over the fence and into the field. I soon discovered that a sand wedge is the ideal club for chipping teabags back into a dustbin, and a seven iron gave just the right height and distance when dealing with such sundries as a toilet roll tube, eggshells or the top off a low-calorie salad cream bottle. The best bit of all was the pickled onion from down the side of the settee. It was perhaps the nearest thing to a golfball that I had found all afternoon, and it was a challenge in that my backswing would be impeded by a kitten's backside.

I consulted the rule book and found that I was allowed to move this off-white obstacle with the bright yellow chin, and so I picked him up and swung him round due east. He didn't even know he'd been moved, and together we spent a most pleasant half hour as he worked away at his custard and I attempted to chip the pickled onion back into the bin.

Then a voice behind me said. 'Shall I come back in ten minutes, or shall we leave it for this week?'

I think I was slightly more embarrassed than the kitten until the dustbin man said, 'What's that over there?'

He strolled over to a pert little beetroot perched cheekily on the rockery and I could have kicked myself for missing it.

'What do you think – a nine iron?'

'Should be about right,' I said, 'as long as you keep the face open.' I have no idea what that means, but somebody once said it to me.

We chipped away happily for some time – he with his beetroot, me with my pickled onion – until, with Jacklinesque precision, his beetroot sailed right into the heart of the dustbin.

'Game, set and match,' he said as he heaved the dustbin on to his shoulder. I picked up my golfbag and we strolled up the drive, the kitten at our heels.

'I nearly chucked him in the crusher last week – he

was hiding in a bin liner. Little sod, he is – that reminds me, how's the wife?'

'Not too good at the moment,' I told him, 'but she seems to be pulling round.'

The kitten jumped into the boot just as I was about to hurl in the clubs.

'She'll be all right. Fighter your wife, got nine lives she has – just like him.'

I hoped he was right, but silently I wondered just how many the pair of them had used up already.

19

Diana sounded much brighter on the phone. The voice was alive, and for the first time she wanted to know what was going on at home. She had been in the National a month now and it had been good for her – it was a hospital for grown-ups, where patients were talked to and not at.

The sister shouted down the phone.

'Would you mind cutting this conversation short – there are three men sitting on your wife's bed and they're becoming restless.'

'Do me a favour,' said Diana, 'bring me my watch when you come down – it's with my jewellery.'

'OK.'

'On second thoughts, forget it.'

'It's no trouble.'

'No – don't worry. It'll only finish up in dew-drop's locker over there.'

'Whatever you say.'

'And don't worry about these three fellas – we're only talking about sex.'

So that was all right, then.

I was very good. I boiled myself an egg and cut two slices of toast into soldiers before I rushed upstairs and opened the jewellery drawer. She had changed her mind too quickly about the watch – there was something in the drawer she didn't want me to see.

It took me about a minute to find the second cache of Soneryl hidden in an empty lipstick case by the side of the watch – there were fifteen of the pink tablets this time, and they spilled across the surface of the dressing table, hiding behind hairbrushes and ring-trees, doing their best to preserve Diana's secret. I had searched the bedroom twice before without success. There were so many possible hiding places and so many bits and pieces. Still – two down, one to go. I counted the tablets once more before screwing the polythene bag back into the case, and felt so very sad that they should be there at all and yet more than a little smug with myself for having found them, as I sat down in front of the television with my tray on my knee.

My egg was past its best, but I still might have finished it had not James Herriot, in living colour, rolled up his sleeve, greased his arm to the elbow and then shoved it right up a cow's backside. Should a smug little smile ever dare to flicker across my face, it will live for only a few seconds before being wiped away. This time, however, I had the cow for company.

The Passmores officially took over the factory, and the Midland Bank patted me on the head with one hand and took the money off me with the other.

'At least you'll have more time for your writing,' my mother told me as she ironed her overall. I had never seen anyone, not even my mother, iron a garment whilst still wearing it – but she did.

'Saves getting the ironing board out – can't be bothered with it.'

She pressed the sides of the unbuttoned front on the table and then spot-ironed the sleeves, touching the iron against her arm. The back she ignored – she wouldn't be able to see the back.

'You've missed a bit.'

She touched up a crease against her thigh, and then I winced as she confidently ironed both lapels, the handle against her cheek.

'That's very dangerous.'

'Not if you know what you're doing.'

We sat and ate fish and chips. Twice a week since Diana had been in London – Wednesdays and Fridays – I had brought in fish and chips, and my mother was always delighted and completely surprised.

'Oh, that's lovely – I wasn't expecting this,' and then she would hand me the two dinner plates warming by the fire and reach for the vinegar bottle standing ready on the mantelpiece.

The television would be switched on, but the sound would be muted so that we could have a nice long chat.

'Diana's coming home on Saturday.'

'I *am* glad – it's been a long time.'

Whisky sat on the arm of the settee and became increasingly irritated with my mother, who offered him only chips, so he jumped down and sat on my foot – the softer touch. I gave him a piece of fish and he dribbled it under the settee. My mother pointed to the television where a dozen ostriches were strutting across an African plain. Playing around their feet were thirty or forty baby ostriches.

'They're extinct, you know,' my mother told me, and I wondered if the birds were aware of this fact. Perhaps it was better if they weren't.

'What they should do,' she declared, pointing her knife at the set, 'is send someone out with a camera to film all the animals that are extinct.'

It seemed an appropriate point at which to ask the question.

'Do you remember the sleeping tablets you used to have – the Soneryl?'

'Yes.'

'Did you ever give any to Diana?'

'She had fifty – just in case.'

'In case of what?'

'Same reason as I've got some tucked away – just in case.'

Like most people, I had my views on euthanasia. I was in favour of a gentle escape from pain, if that's all there was to be – I had put forward my views with some confidence at parties after a glass or two of wine.

294

But when reality creeps in it fudges the edges of our beliefs and shows us how trite our words can be when put to the test – I didn't want Diana to become extinct.

The southern branch of the family had rallied round and made sure that Diana had never been short of visitors. Joyce and David had travelled up from the Isle of Wight, Vera had driven in from Hampshire, and Roy, Ian and Dee had pushed the wheelchair around London when Maggie, Chris and Helen were exhausted. Gareth, her fellow patient, had spent hours with her – talking through the problems in his young life. He had been temporarily discharged, even though he was still very ill, but nevertheless he had travelled all the way up from Herne Bay to see her.

Sally had been the mortar in this wall of visitors and Diana had thrived on the company, but now, as she lay on her bed at home, she was exhausted. However, she always put on a show when visitors called. It was as though she was on stage – the collapse would come as the curtain fell.

'She's much better today, isn't she?'

'She's doing very well,' I would agree, and then go upstairs to help put the pieces together again.

It was the physiotherapy that had drained her in the National. She had decided to give it another try, but any benefit she had derived from the well-meant exercises had bled her of energy until she was unable even to sit up in the car on the way home and I had curled her tight on the back seat, packed in with coats and blankets.

Nothing new had been brought to light in the hospital, but the specialist, Professor Thomas, had kept his promise and talked to her at length before she left. This was so important – so many times she had been allowed to dissolve from the scene as though the specialist, having nothing to declare, was washing his hands of her.

'There's really nothing more we can do at the moment – it's all a bit of a mystery.'

'I didn't expect you to find anything.'

'If your condition deteriorates – then we could try again.'

'Thank you.'

For the next two months we existed. Day and night seemed very much the same, with the heavy bedroom curtains closed to shut out the light that hurt her eyes, and the house itself felt like a tomb as I padded around barefoot so as not to disturb the funereal peace.

Sleep sat lightly upon her and I guarded, very closely, those moments when she could sink into oblivion. The phone was taken off the hook and at eight-thirty one morning I found myself out on the road, dragging a driver from his car after he had chosen to lean on his horn rather than knock on the front door of his intended passenger.

'You selfish bastard!'

'I didn't think.'

'Well, try it now and then – it doesn't hurt.'

I like to think that I apologized because I was wrong and not because he was a foot and half taller and three stone heavier than I was.

The ice cream van seemed to wait around the corner until she slept, and then it would advance with a ragged version of the 'Teddy Bears' Picnic' blasting from a tinny speaker, but I had learnt my lesson.

If anything I slept less than she did. When she was awake I was needed, and whilst she was asleep I rode shotgun and kept the natives at bay.

My mind was becoming muddy and my thinking fuddled. Small matters took on immense proportions – not being able to find the top off a jar of pickled onions would bring with it a ridiculous despair that would depress me even further when I found the lid that night, tucked away in my trouser pocket. I found myself talking to Nick in a whisper so as not to wake her – in the middle of the Fine Fare supermarket we were, with Diana asleep in bed a mile away.

Every week I turned in five or six humorous pieces for the BBC and the odd magazine, and they would chart my chaotic domestic life with all the bones removed for easy listening. They were very popular.

'Dear Mr Longden, I loved the story where you

painted your office walls and ceiling with gloss paint, thinking it was emulsion. It was very funny – I bet it looked like a butcher's shop, just as you said. You must be very absent-minded. Did it really take six coats of emulsion to cover it?'

'Dear Mrs A, Thank you for your letter – it's good to know that someone is listening. Yes, it happened just as I said. I thought it was hard going with the roller, but my mind was elsewhere....'

I didn't tell her that I sat down on the floor next morning and cried at my stupidity – that's not part of the bargain.

The months rolled by and autumn came, and with it a break in the clouds.

'I'm sick of bread and milk.'

'And I'm sick of making it – what would you like?'

'Smoked salmon sandwiches – thin ones with the crusts cut off.'

'How about a beefburger?'

'That'll do.'

We had another go at Stephen King's *Firestarter* – this time I read it aloud to her, and frightened the life out of both of us. We were also largely responsible for the video boom in this country, as I brought them home from the shop in armfuls. The pause button was put on overtime as Diana blacked out on average three times a film. It took us a week to get through *Dune*, which made it, as far as we were concerned, the most cost-effective video of all time.

But mostly we talked. Diana sitting up, muffled in pillows, with me perched on the edge of the bed, and between us the embroidery that was nearing completion. I knew more about the back of this picture than I did the front. I was in charge of the more intricate work – such as threading needles and plucking tiny beads from small brown jars and holding her forefinger and thumb together so that the needle wouldn't fall. I held the frame steady and, after Diana had selected her mark, I pushed the needle through the padded gold and burgundy kid. I was grossly underpaid. She selected a length of gold wire and handed it to me for threading.

'I forgot to ask you – did you find them?'

'Find what?'

'The sleeping tablets – in my jewellery drawer.'

'Yes – I put them back again.'

She took the needle from me and worked a delicate web around an island of beads.

'That was nice of you. It's not that I'm trying to keep you out – it's just that I need to be in charge of something. I couldn't take another ten or twenty years of this, and I want to be able to decide when I've had enough.'

I cut some loose threads from the back of the picture and then loaded the needle once more.

'I understand – I really do – but can't you see that I

don't want to just walk into the bedroom one day and find you gone? Every time I come home I run up the stairs, and if you're asleep it frightens the life out of me. If it's going to happen, I want time to say goodbye – properly.'

She laid the picture on the bed and took my hand.

'Don't you see? If you helped me and they found out – you could go to prison . . .'

'It's hardly likely.'

'. . . and I don't think you could handle the guilt.'

From time to time my mind stood aside and wondered how we could talk so calmly about such a thing.

'Have you found the other tablets?'

'I found the shoe polish tin.'

'Bloody hell! I thought that was a master stroke. Is that it – that and the lipstick?'

'Yes.'

She tried to pick up the frame, and I took it from her and held it steady so that she could work.

'Do me a favour – don't look for the others. Leave it as my secret, and I promise to talk it through with you before I do anything.'

'I promise.'

She speared a small red bead with the needle and her small pink tongue poked out between her lips as she concentrated. She saw me watching her.

'And stop worrying – I'm not going anywhere until I've finished this bloody thing.'

★

It was finished within the week, and she displayed it proudly to me as though I had never seen it before.

'You see, the beads are supposed to be tumbling there.'

'It's lovely.'

'And that's sequin waste – pretty, isn't it?'

'Very pretty.'

'It's the best I can do. I'm a bit limited.'

'I think it's wonderful.'

'Then hold it the right way up.'

The next day we had planned to have a day on the town. The Hallamshire in the morning to see Fred at the Plaster Unit, and an hour with Pat Harvey on the way home. In between, if all went well, we would fit in a little light shopping in Sheffield – Coles, perhaps, where the lifts were roomy and the aisles were wide.

But as the night wore on it became plain that tomorrow would be just another day that drifted away from us. Twice during the night I had filled the bath with hot water and Diana had soaked her body to ease the pain, but nothing would touch it this time, and then her hands had clawed and a migraine completed the misery.

It was six in the morning before she fell asleep. Her leg was cold as ice, and I lay by the side of her and tried to warm it with mine. After half an hour it was as though I had frostbite from the knee down, and I substituted myself with a hot water bottle and crept downstairs in search of the fan heater and a cup of tea. I slept for a couple of hours or so on the hearthrug, and then crept back upstairs to get dressed.

At first I thought Diana was asleep – her nose peeped over the sheets but her eyes were closed as I fumbled under the covers for the hot water bottle which would be cold by now. I found it – it was still warm, but the leg was frozen and it chilled the surrounding sheets.

As I withdrew the bottle gently from its nest I looked up and saw her eyes smiling at me, a weary smile that would be too tired to take in the lips.

'Am I being interfered with?'

I produced the hot water bottle with a magician's flourish.

'Oh – pity. I wouldn't know, I can't feel a thing down there.'

'Breakfast first, then I shall anoint you with exotic oils.'

'Bath first – sorry, but I need one.'

I filled the bath and squeezed the last drop from the bottle of moisturizing foam. We used gallons of the stuff – I had thought of asking Marks & Spencer's if they could organize delivery by tanker.

The towels were still wet from last night's dip, and I fetched clean ones from the airing cupboard.

'All ready.'

Still just her nose peeped over the sheets, but now the smile had gone from her eyes.

'I need a little longer – it hurts too much to move.'

'No hurry. I'll stick these towels in the washer.'

Down in the kitchen I stuffed the machine to the gunnels, topping it off with two rather disgusting oven gloves. It paid to keep an eye on the washer – it had a mind of its own. If it was packed wrongly it would wait five minutes and then, when it thought you weren't looking, it would belt across the kitchen floor and make a break for it off up the drive. I dried a few pots and pans and kept a weather eye open, but for once it behaved itself – perhaps the oven gloves were keeping it occupied.

Time to see if Diana could make it now – there was no more hot water, and we couldn't afford to let the bath go too cold.

The bed was empty. I hadn't heard her get up, but then the washing machine made a hell of a din. She must be in the toilet.

I posted myself outside the toilet door. I wished she wouldn't do this – she could cling to the furniture in the bedroom, but the no man's land at the top of the stairs was dangerous and she would perform her double axel with triple pike once too often. I slid my bottom down the wall and sat on the carpet, chin on knees, and waited. She needed privacy, and if she needed help she would ask.

But she didn't ask – it was too quiet. I knocked on the door.

303

'Diana?'

No answer. I opened the door – she wasn't there. The bathroom. She must be in the bathroom.

I pushed open the door, and at first the room seemed empty. And then I saw her – she was lying face down in the bath, one foot curled over the rim, her hair swimming.

As I moved towards her the foot unhooked itself and slid down into the bath. I put my arms underneath her and tried to lift her out, but her body jackknifed and then slid out of my grasp. Her head, you idiot! Get her head out of the water. I grabbed her under the arms and lifted, but she was made of rubber and the head dipped back into the foam.

Still holding her, I jumped into the bath and tried to turn her over. She wouldn't move. Christ! I was standing on her hand. I knelt down so that I could take hold properly, but she was slippery with the foam and, as I raised her, I could feel her oozing out of my arms again. My feet went from under me and we fell together, her head crashing against the taps. Oh God, I've hurt her – please don't let me make a mess of this. I was trying to be too gentle. Just get her out.

With my knees and arms I lifted her once more, and with a final heave bundled her over the side and on to the floor. She lay where she fell, still and silent, her nightdress clinging wet around her knees, a trickle of water escaping from her lips.

I climbed out of the bath and took hold of her. I

didn't know what to do – I didn't bloody well know what to do. Should I turn her on her face or on her side? Why didn't I know these things – why did I never listen?

I turned her face down, her head to one side, and began to pump and press as I thought I remembered having seen it done in a film once. It seemed awkward, and nothing was happening. I pumped and pumped, and then I turned her on her side and tried again.

Maybe if she had blacked out she hadn't taken in much water. The kiss of life! I took a deep breath and put my mouth to hers – nothing. I was wasting time – oh, God, what should I do?

I ran into the bedroom and dialled 999. I can't remember what I said – the girl seemed very calm.

I covered Diana with a towel, and then lifted her head and cradled her in my lap. She must have had a blackout and fallen in the bath – but the nightdress was around her knees. Was she taking it off? She would have had to step out of it – she couldn't use her arms above her head. Had she just fallen? Please, God – let her have had a blackout.

What was I doing just sitting here? Come on, do something – she needs you. Once again I tried to breathe life into her, but I was crying and I couldn't seem to get any air. So I sat and held her in my arms – I was useless.

Someone was knocking on the front door. I laid Diana's head gently on the floor and raced downstairs. I flung the door open – two men stood there.

'Up here.'

I was on the landing and they weren't following me. I turned and shouted.

'She's up here.'

A man in a suit appeared at the bottom of the stairs.

'Mr Longden? Customs and Excise – we would like to see your books.'

'Not now.'

'You've had a letter, Mr Longden,' said another voice.

'I can't – not now.'

'With the accountant, are they?'

One of them laughed, and then there was a commotion in the hall and two ambulance men brushed them aside and climbed the stairs towards me.

I reached the bathroom first, but one held me back at the door as the other went through to Diana.

I watched as the man knelt over her. He had equipment – I don't know what it was. He did something with it – I don't know what he did. I do know that he looked up at me and shook his head.

'Come on,' said his partner. 'Let's go downstairs,' and he put his arm around me and I walked away and left my wife lying dead on the bathroom floor.

20

The room was full of people and they were being very nice to me. The ambulance men called me Deric and suggested we ring Nick. How did he know about Nick? I looked at him for the first time and recognized him – it was Jo's uncle. What was his name? It's very rude to forget someone's name.

Dr MacFarlane went straight upstairs and I moved to follow him, but the policeman suggested that I should wait. There were two policemen – one was young and one wasn't.

'Let's put the kettle on,' said the ambulance man, and I asked who took sugar and followed him into the kitchen. It was a very good cup of tea. Sometimes you make a cup and it's wonderful – sometimes it's just a cup of tea. This one was very good and I shouldn't be enjoying it so much – Diana was dead.

Dr MacFarlane came downstairs and said how sorry he was and that he would call back and see me. The older policeman walked with him up the drive and the younger one pulled his chair closer towards the hearth where I was squatting.

'Do you feel like telling us what happened?'

'I'll just go and see Diana first.'

The ambulance man – Godfrey, that was it, Godfrey Bettis – Godfrey didn't think it was a very good idea.

'You drink your tea, Deric – my friend's looking after Diana.'

The older policeman came back and I told them what had happened and how useless I had been. They listened and they asked me questions and they told me that I wasn't useless – but then they hadn't been there.

'Nobody could have done anything,' Godfrey was saying. 'It was too late – finish your tea.'

I took a mouthful – it was cold and tasted like straw. The others didn't have tea – why was that?

'Would you like to change your clothes?' the older policeman asked me. I moved my feet and they squelched – I was wet through.

I took my shoes off and then my socks.

'I trod on her hand,' I told them, and then Nick came through the door and put his arms around me.

They took Diana away to the ambulance. They hurried past the open door in the hall before I knew what was happening – Nick said it was for the best.

Michael Jackson came over from across the road and explained what would happen now – there would be an inquest. He was a Chief Inspector and he was very kind – seeing my blank expression, he came back the next day and told me again.

★

There was a vast emptiness about the house, almost as though it were hollow, and Nick and I began to tidy up, clean the ashtrays, wash the pots – anything to restore normality.

'I knew she was gone, Dad – as soon as I got the message to ring home.'

'We must tell Sally.'

'We can't just ring her.'

'We'll go and fetch her.'

I needed to change, but I couldn't go upstairs – not yet. Nick anticipated me.

'I'll get you some clothes.'

He disappeared once again as I pulled on the jeans and sweater, and then I heard the bathwater gush.

He came downstairs and fell on his knees in front of the fire, his face buried in his hands – now it was my turn to be strong for a while.

We called at my mother's and told her. She sat down at the table, tears running down her cheeks.

'I bought her a nightie – I'm supposed to pick it up today.'

We stayed for an hour, and just before we left she took me in to the kitchen. At that stage, only my mother could have got away with telling me, 'Perhaps it's for the best.'

Nick drove, and the M1 seemed to go on forever. We talked about Diana – dredging for happy memories.

'You'll never believe this, Dad.'

'Try me.'

'I didn't want to think as I drove home from Nottingham, so I put the radio on very loud.'

When Nick switched on the radio his car bounced.

'I was just passing Mum's old shop in Matlock Bath, and Simon Bates played "Wide Eyed and Legless". I had to stop – I couldn't see for tears.'

Sally was delighted to see us. She moved to throw her arms around me and then stopped – her eyes searching first mine and then Nick's.

'No . . .'

'I'm sorry, darling.'

With a cry she ran back into her room and fell on the bed. She sobbed, her body shaking, and Nick and I joined in although we were nearly cried out now.

I made a pot of vile tea and tried to make conversation with a strange young man who sat on his bike in the kitchen.

Sally perched on the edge of her bed now, and with Nick's arms around her she dried out and passed into that empty aching space that Nick and I were coming to know so well.

That night I rang my mother to see if all was well with her. It wasn't but she put on a brave face.

'I've just had a good stand-up wash – life must go on.'

I gave my hands and face a lick at the kitchen sink – she wouldn't have approved, but I couldn't go into the bathroom.

The embroidery was lying on the bed and I held it on my knee and traced the stitches with my finger.

'I'm not going anywhere until I've finished this bloody thing.'

There were several bottles of beads on the bedside table – she used old medicine bottles, of which she had an endless supply. I began to tuck them back neatly in her sewing box – I had nothing better to do, but I didn't have Diana's knack. I took them all out and started again. One bottle was bigger than the others, and I put it on one side and then forgot about it.

It was still there in the morning, nudging up against the alarm clock. I picked it up and read the label: 'Mrs A. M. Longden Soneryl 60 tablets, take one at night.'

She hadn't needed them after all.

There seemed so much to do, and yet it was all done so quickly – the experts took over, and then it was a matter of waiting for the funeral.

Life took on a surreal quality. The house had lost all its warmth – it was full of strange furniture that wasn't very comfortable. There was a sense of being on holiday with the kids in a dingy boarding house and we were killing time, waiting for the rain to stop.

'Put the radio on if you want, Sally.'

'No, it's all right.'

There were so many phone calls to make, and we took it in turns. When we weren't making calls, the phone rang.

I struggled desperately with my guilt – every time I closed my eyes the scene in the bathroom was there on the screen. My helplessness – my stupidity.

I tried so hard to come to terms with it, to keep it from the children – they wouldn't know about guilt. But it twisted and turned until my mind was bruised and for the hundredth time.

'If only I had . . . .'

Nick stopped me before I could tell them yet again.

'Dad! The day before Mum died I was coming up to see her – but there was a football match on the television, so I watched that instead.'

I had no monopoly on guilt.

Friends came to the door in waves – some could handle it, others couldn't.

Paul Wolfenden could – he sat on the settee and talked about Diana. So many callers found it difficult to mention her name. Paul talked about her for hours – about the early days of the double act when we made her join in.

'Do you remember Stirling? And that time in Skegness?'

We remembered other times and soon we were

laughing, the four of us, as Diana's spirit came flooding back into the room.

It was a beautiful day for November. The bright sunshine gave the illusion of warmth, and it was the sort of day Diana would have loved.

Nick had gone to fetch my mother, and the cars would be here soon – was there anything I had forgotten? Janet, Diana's sister, was having the family back at her house in Bakewell afterwards – I was grateful, it was something I didn't have to think about and I wanted the house quiet. I should need a bolthole after the funeral.

Dorothy, Diana's twin sister, had rung from the States earlier and cried because she couldn't come over – she had problems with her back, which gave us pause for thought.

The door opened and my mother burst in – she wore the blue hat she had bought for Nick's wedding, and she seemed to have shrunk. She looked older somehow and her eyes were tired, but she was determined to be the matriarchal rock. If she sensed the merest suspicion of silence coming on, she felt that it was her duty in life to fill it. Today there were many holes for her to cap.

She took in the scene at a glance and nudged me in the ribs.

'Where's the spread?'

'The what?'

'The food – where's the food?'

'They're all going back to Janet's.'

She was happy now – she had a mission and she moved amongst the guests.

'We're all going back to Janet's afterwards – there will be food at Janet's.'

She told Janet, who thanked her for letting her know. At my father's funeral those business friends of his who didn't know her had paid their respects to a tearful Nellie Elliot and mistaken my mother for the caterer. She dealt with grief in her own way – she was a lovely woman.

She found the going harder in the car. Nick and Jo, Sally and I were a tough audience, and apart from the odd, 'I can remember when all this was fields,' she admitted defeat and sank reluctantly into the tearful silence.

I had dreaded this moment. All through the week I had made decisions as though in a dream.

'Now, Mr Longden – about the coffin?'

'Have you given any thought to the hymns, Mr Longden?'

It wasn't for real. I was an actor speaking lines in rehearsal for a play that would never take place – not for a long time, anyway. But the days had ground by and the time had come and I wasn't ready for it.

The car passed through large gates and into a driveway and my mother shuddered.

'It's an awful word – crematorium. Why don't they call them something else?'

We drove past flower beds and lawns towards a wooden awning and the main doors. People gathered outside – lots of people, in large groups. They were wearing hats and smart suits, and they stopped talking and turned towards the car as we approached.

'We're too early,' Nick voiced with some concern. 'There's another funeral.'

But the driver kept going until he came to a gentle halt beneath the awning. Men in black with solemn faces opened the car doors and we stepped out.

The crowd had moved in behind the car and were standing, watching. I recognized a face, and then another and another – they *were* here to see Diana. Why hadn't they gone in? What had gone wrong?

My mother crumpled slightly and Sally and I each took an arm – and then music played and the doors were opened and I found myself walking through into the chapel.

It was packed to the rafters – they lined the walls and stood at the back, and those with seats rose in waves as we walked down the aisle. My mother looked bewildered and hesitated slightly – we tightened our grip on her and walked slowly forward, towards the only empty pew in the chapel.

That's why they were waiting outside – they couldn't get in.

'*Deric – do you think many people will turn up at my funeral?*'

315

The tears flooded down my cheeks, but the joy in my heart was such that I thought it might burst.

We knelt and then sat down. As I raised my eyes I saw the coffin resting on a dais – it looked very new and rather lonely. There were no flowers to decorate the shining wood, just a simple wreath and, standing proudly to one end, the little red hat with its feathers ruffling and its veil modestly downcast.

Sally put her hand on my arm and laid her head on my shoulder and whispered.

'Doesn't she look beautiful?'

She did – so very beautiful.

Ian Gregory stood at the lectern and cleared his throat. We had known Ian for years, first as a newspaperman and then as a BBC news reporter – at last he had gone straight and was now a Congregational Minister. He was talking to us.

'Deric made Diana a promise. Firstly she wanted the pop song "Wide Eyed and Legless" played at her funeral – she thought it appropriate since she spent most of her time in a wheelchair and yet still, rather cleverly, she managed to fall downstairs with alarming regularity . . .'

There were audible smiles all around us – they knew her well, and then Ian's rich voice went on.

' . . .we tried, but somehow it wasn't the same without Andy Fairweather-Lowe to sing it for us – we couldn't find it in the hymn book, either.'

This time the smiles were louder, and somehow the feeling spread throughout the chapel that we were here, not simply to mourn, but to celebrate a triumph.

'Deric made her another promise. She bought only two hats in her life – one for her honeymoon and the other for Nick's wedding. She loved that wedding hat and often Deric would find her sitting up in bed, wearing a nightie and watching television – the hat perched on her head. She insisted that, at her funeral, the hat be placed on her coffin, and as you can see she is wearing it today.'

Still the tears ran down our faces, but somehow the coffin no longer seemed to be the embodiment of doom. She had no pain now and she was wearing her hat.

'I want Ian Gregory to conduct the service – I think he likes me.'

'I think he does, love – and he's doing you proud.'

The hymns were sung with vigour – no thin piping from a handful of voices. They were belted out in celebration.

Nick reached across the front of me to take a tissue from Sally, but my mother spirited it away from him and blew her nose. Ian was drawing to a close.

'We are all infinitely more human for knowing Diana than otherwise we would have been. Because of her we can laugh and cry with confidence. And

317

because we shall not forget her, we will be able to face up to the future with the courage she taught us, the fun she shared with us, and one more thing of untold value – a definition of beauty, which, had we not known her, we could not have understood.'

As we stepped outside into the November sun I saw the flowers for the first time – bank upon bank of them, spilling over the grass verges and down on to the paths.

And then there were the people – hundreds of them. Some were friends we saw every week, others perhaps once a year. There were those I didn't recognize, and I wanted to meet and talk to each and every one of them.

Sally said later that I took off like a headless chicken, diving in amongst them, hugging and shaking hands – I wanted to share this moment with those who had caught just a glimpse of the woman whom I had loved with all my heart. They talked of her and told me things I didn't know – of the times she had touched their lives.

A young girl waited as we moved towards the car. She stepped forward and took my arm.

'I shampooed Diana's hair whenever you brought her down to the salon. I don't get on very well with my parents, and when things got too bad at home I used to look in the appointments book and see when she was coming in. Then I'd save it all up and pour it all out to her while I washed her hair – she always

318

used to listen and tell me what to do. I shan't half miss her.'

Janet came over and waited until the girl had finished, then she asked me: 'Are you going home now, Deric?'

'I don't think so – I'll come over to Bakewell with you.'

I didn't need the bolthole now – I wanted to be with friends.

Some time later I walked into the chemist's in Smedley Street and Margaret called me into the dispensary.

'I don't know if you're ready for this.'

'For what?'

She took a deep breath – whatever it was, it was going to take some telling.

'I knew Diana had died, long before you told me.'

'How?'

'That afternoon a policeman came into the shop – he was only young. He said he needed to sit down, he'd just come from the mortuary.'

I sat down – *I* wasn't sure if I was ready for this.

'He said he'd just seen a beautiful young woman lying there. He was used to seeing people who had died – but this woman took his breath away.'

She was looking at me to see how I was taking it – I was taking it pretty well, I thought.

'Then he asked me if I knew a Diana Longden – I couldn't believe that she could be dead.'

I blinked and Margaret swallowed, and then she went on.

'He said he couldn't take his eyes off her because the strange thing was – there didn't seem to be a damn thing wrong with her.'

Diana would have loved that.